TABLE OF CONTENTS

- Central Nervous System
- immune system
- Human Body Diagram
- Parts of Tongue
- Parts of Stomach
- Parts of Hand
- Skeletal System
- Human Front Muscles
- Human Back Muscles
- Digestive System
- Parts of Mouth
- Endocrine System
- Urinary System
- Respiratory System
- Parts of Tooth
- Foot Bones
- Mouth & Pharynx
- Parts of Pancreas
- Parts of Leg
- Parts of Skull
- Head & Neck

- MUSCLES OF POSTERIOR VIEW
- MUSCLES OF ANTERIOR VIEW
- HUMAN BACK MUSCLES
- MUSCLES OF THE FACE
- MUSCLES OF THE BODY
- HUMAN FRONT MUSCLES
- MUSCLES OF ANTERIOR FOREARM
- MUSCLES OF POSTERIOR HIP & THIGH
- MUSCLES OF ANTERIOR NECK, SHOULDERS & THORAX
- MUSCLES OF POSTERIOR NECK, SHOULDERS & THORAX
- CLOSER LOOK AT SKELETAL MUSCLES ANATOMY
- MUSCLES OF ANTERIOR HIP & THIGH
- MUSCLES OF LEG(CALF) & FOOT
- MUSCLES OF ANTERIOR ARM & FOREARM
- MUSCLES OF POSTERIOR ARM & FOREARM

ALPHABETS

A - ABDOMEN, ANKLE, ARM, ARMPIT, ARTERY
B - BRAIN, BLADDER, BODY, BELLY, BONES
C - CHEST, CELL, COCCYX, CIRCULATORY SYSTEM
D - DIGESTIVE SYSTEM, DNA, DANDFUL
E - ELBOW, EYE, EARS (AND MANY MORE)

  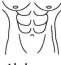

Abdomen   Ankle   Arm   Armpit

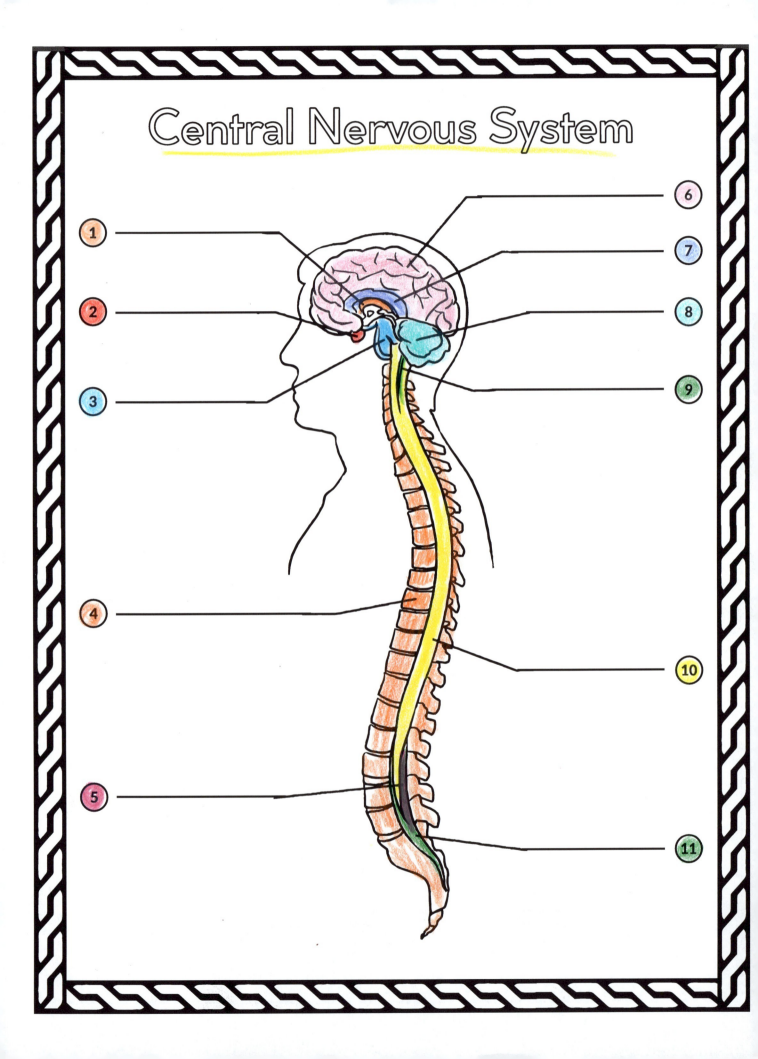

Central Nervous System

(1). Body Of Fornix
(2). Pituitary Gland
(3). Pons Varolii
(4). Vertebral Column
(5). Cauda Equina
(6). Cerebrum
(7). Corpus Callosum
(8). Cerebellum
(9). Brain Stem
(10). Spinal Cord
(11). Dura Mater

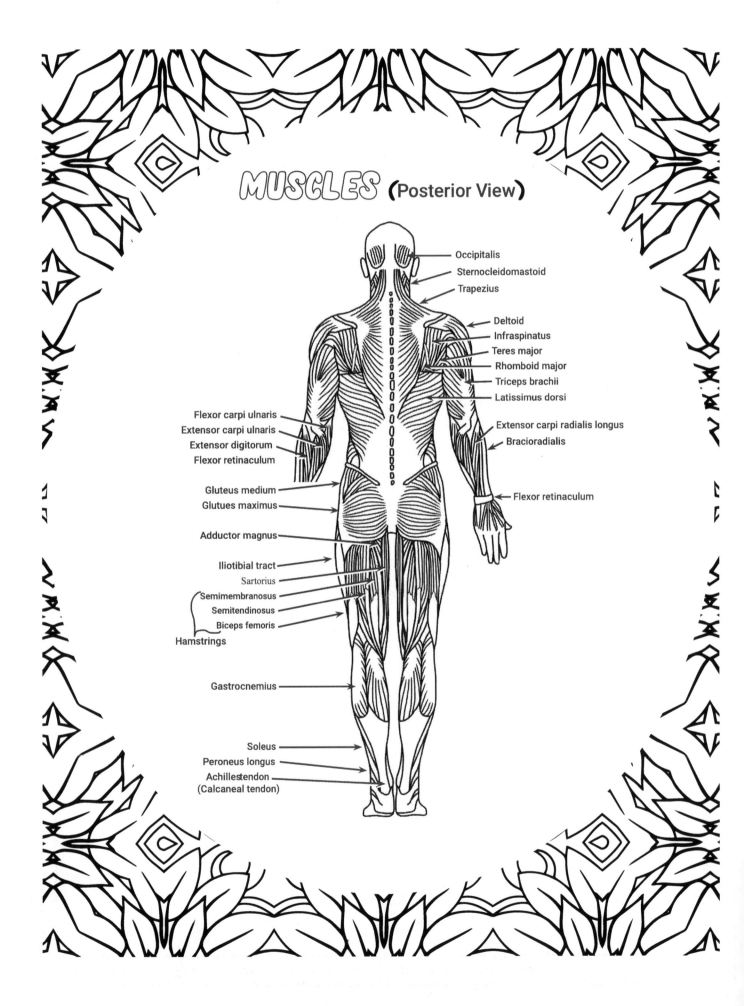

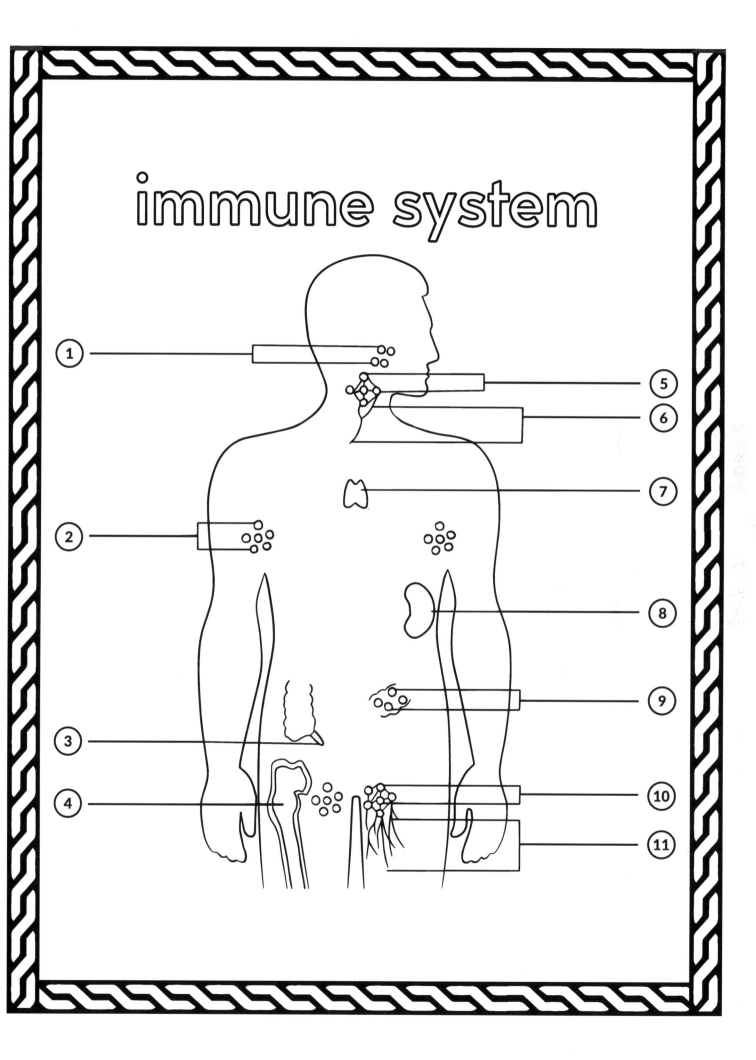

immune system

(1). Tonsils And Adenoids
(2). Lymph Nodes
(3). Appendix
(4). Bone Marrow
(5). Lymph Nodes
(6). Lymphatic Vessels
(7). Thymus
(8). Spleen
(9). Peyer's Patches
(10). Lymph Nodes
(11). Lymphatic Vessels

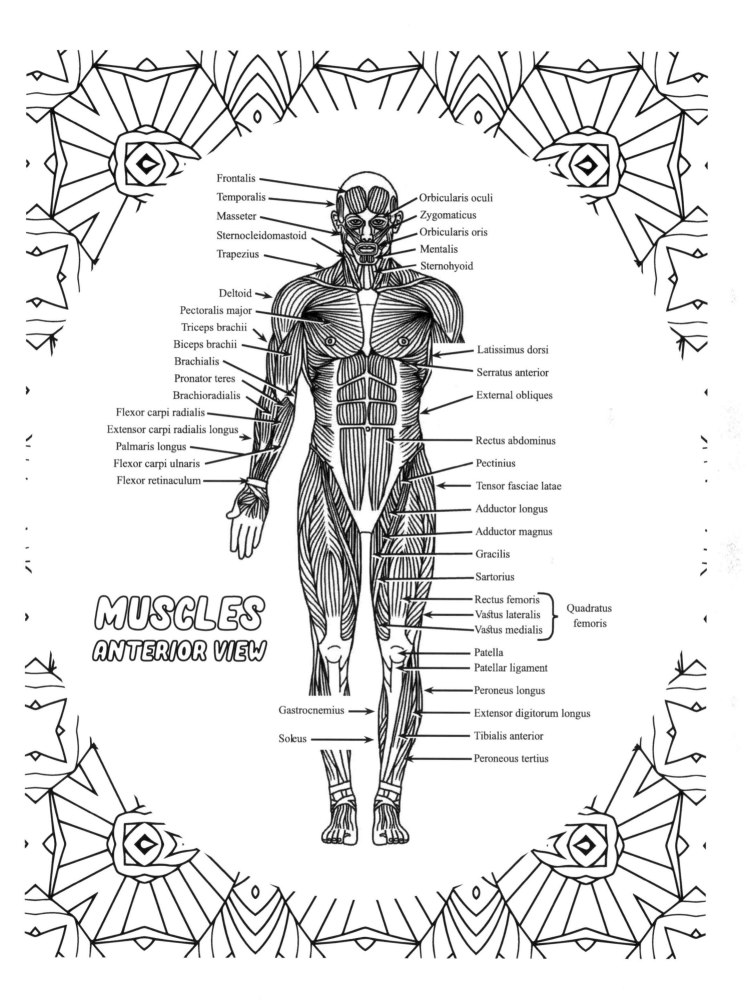

Heart Anatomy

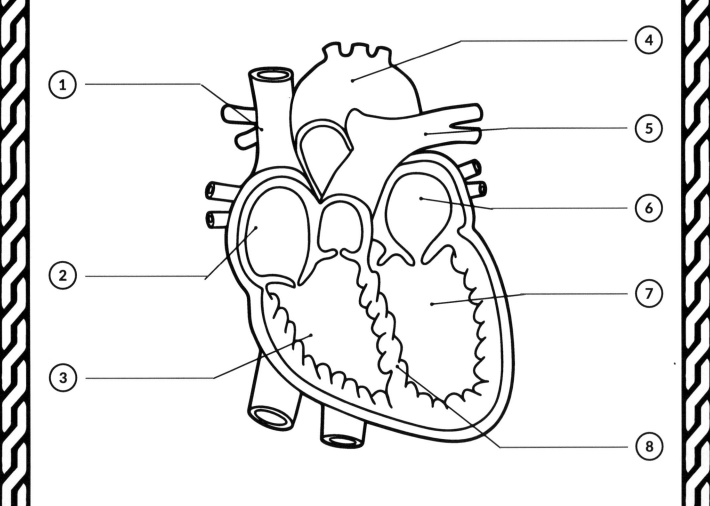

Heart Anatomy

(1). Superior Vena Cava
(2). Right Atrium
(3). Right Ventricle
(4). Aorta
(5). Pulmonary Artery
(6). Left Atrium
(7). Left Ventricle
(8). Interventricular Septum

Liver Anatomy

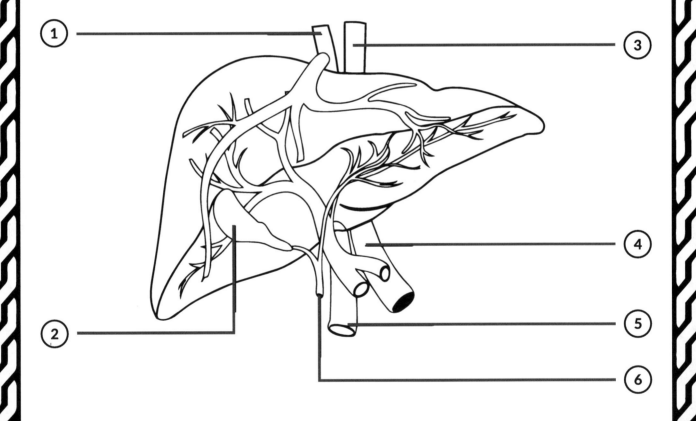

Liver Anatomy

(1). Inferior Vena Cava
(2). Gallbladder
(3). Aorta
(4). Hepatic Artery
(5). Portal Vein
(6). Common Bile Duct

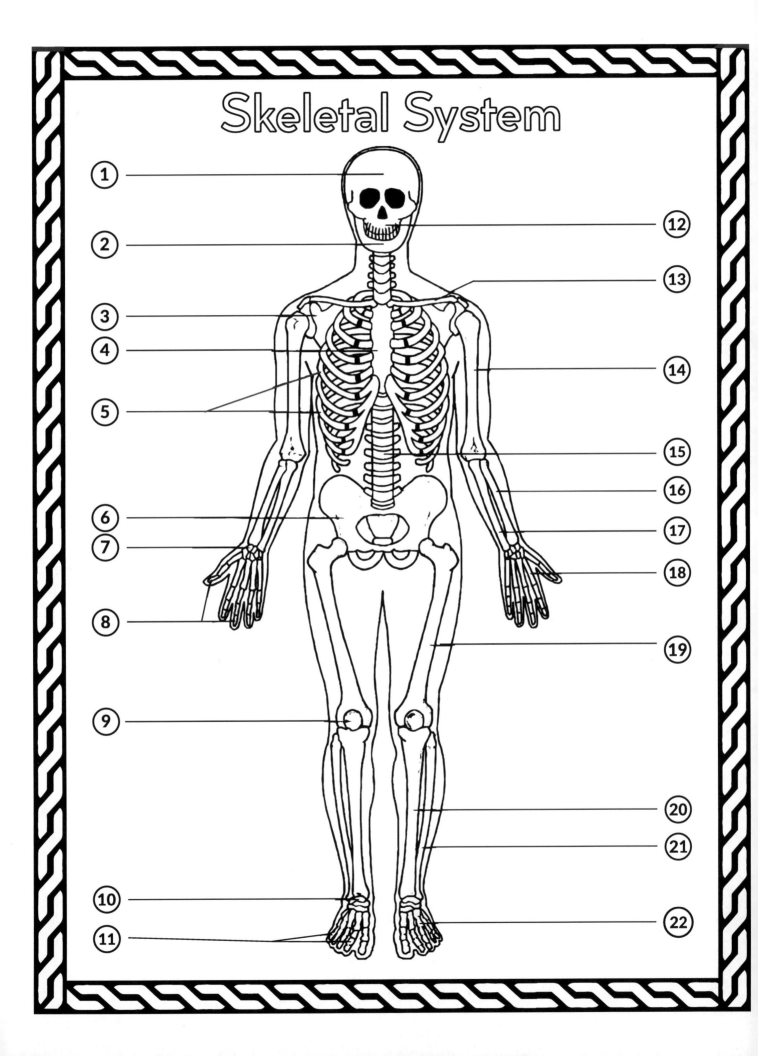

Skeletal System

(1). Cranium
(2). Mandible
(3). Scapula
(4). Sternum
(5). Ribs
(6). Pelvis
(7). Carpals
(8). Phalanges
(9). Patella
(10). Tarsals
(11). Phalanges
(12). Maxilla
(13). Clavicle
(14). Humerus
(15). Vertebral Column
(16). Radius
(17). Ulna
(18). Metacarpals
(19). Femur
(20). Tibia
(21). Fibula
(22). Metatarsals

Mouth Anatomy

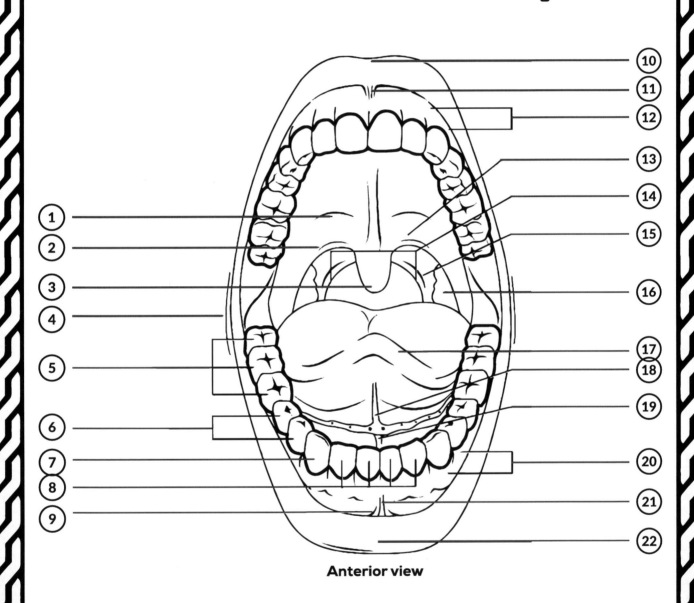

Anterior view

Mouth Anatomy

(1). Hard Palate
(2). Soft Palate
(3). Uvula
(4). Cheek
(5). Molars
(6). Premolars
(7). Cuspid (Canine)
(8). Incisors
(9). Oral Vestibule
(10). Superior Lip
(11). Superior Labial Frenulum
(12). Gingivae (Gums)
(13). Palatoglossal Arch
(14). Fauces
(15). Palatopharyngeal Arch
(16). Palatine Tonsil
(17). Tongue (Underside)
(18). Lingual Frenulum
(19). Opening Duct Of Submandibular Gland
(20). Gingivae (Gums)
(21). Inferior Labial Frenulum
(22). Inferior Lip

Tongue Anatomy

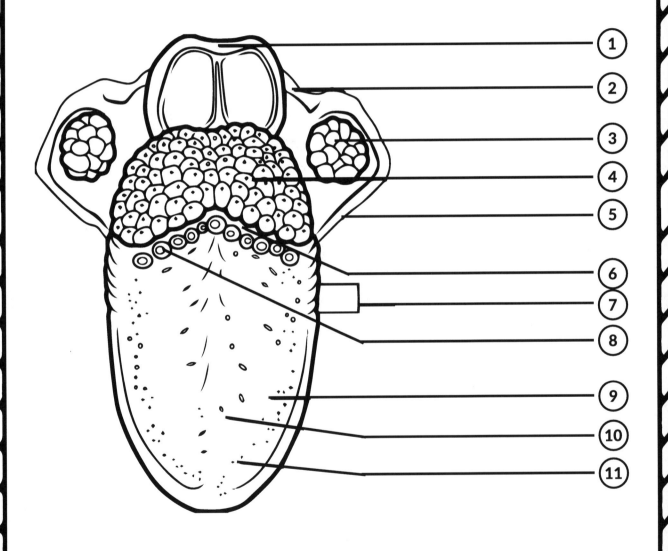

Tongue Anatomy

(1). Epiglottis
(2). Palatopharyngeal Arch
(3). Palatine Tonsil
(4). Lingual Tonsil
(5). Palatoglossal Arch
(6). Terminal Sulcus
(7). Foliate Papillae
(8). Circumvallate Papilla
(9). Dorsum Of Tongue
(10). Fungiform Papilla
(11). Filiform Papilla

Skin Anatomy

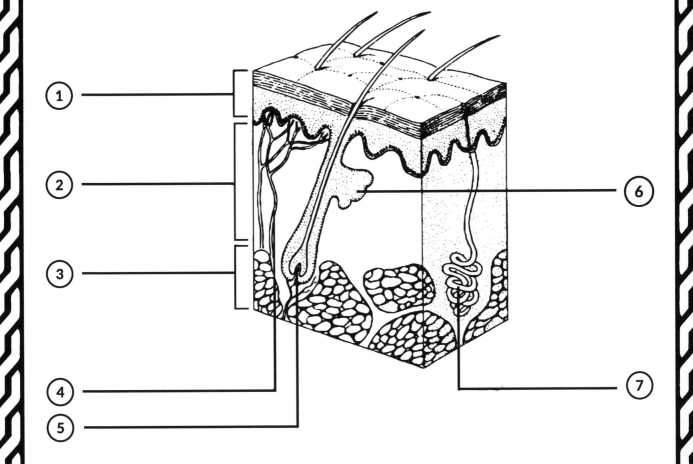

Skin Anatomy

(1). Epidermis
(2). Dermis
(3). Fatty Tissue
(4). Nerve
(5). Follicle
(6). Sweat Gland
(7). Oil Gland

Eye Anatomy

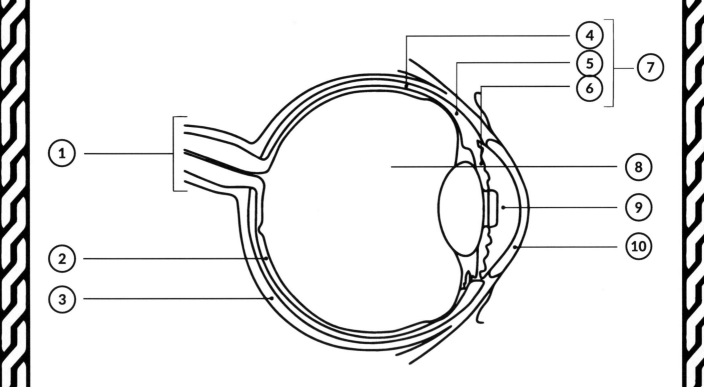

Eye Anatomy

(1). Optic Nerve
(2). Retina
(3). Sclera
(4). Choroid
(5). Ciliary Body
(6). Iris
(7). Uvea
(8). Vitreous
(9). Pupil
(10). Cornea

Skull Anatomy

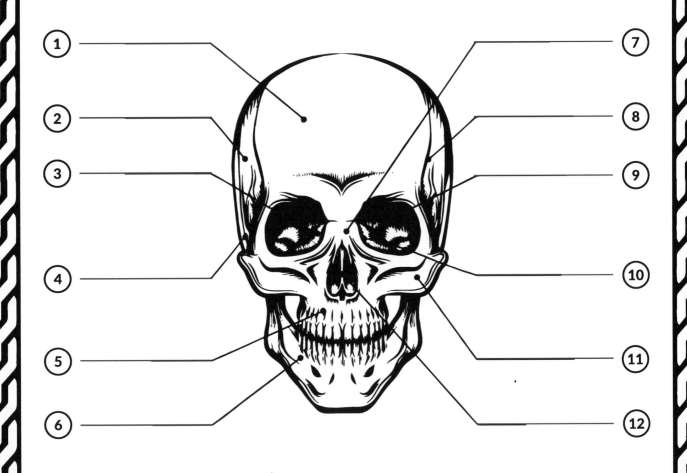

Skull Anatomy

(1). Frontal Bone
(2). Parietal Bone
(3). Ethmoid Bone
(4). Temporal Bone
(5). Maxilla
(6). Mandible
(7). Nasal Bone
(8). Coronal Suture
(9). Sphenoid Bone
(10). Lacrimal Bone
(11). Zygomatic Bone
(12). Vomer

Kidney Anatomy

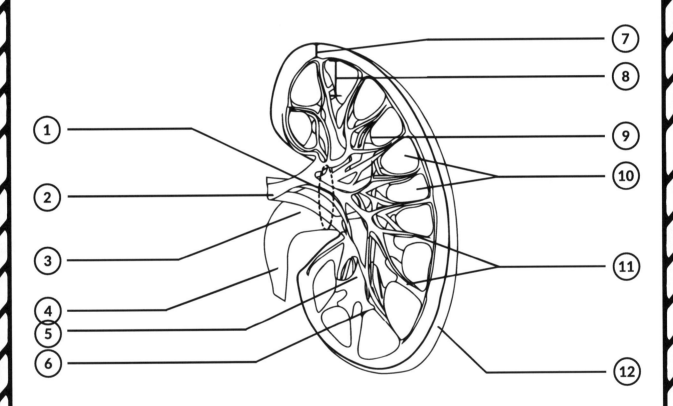

Kidney Anatomy

(1). Hilum
(2). Renal Artery Renal Vein
(3). Renal Pelvis
(4). Ureter
(5). Major Calyx
(6). Minor Calyx
(7). Renal Cortex
(8). Renal Medulla
(9). Renal Papilla
(10). Renal Pyramids
(11). Renal Columns
(12). Fibrous Capsule

Tooth Anatomy

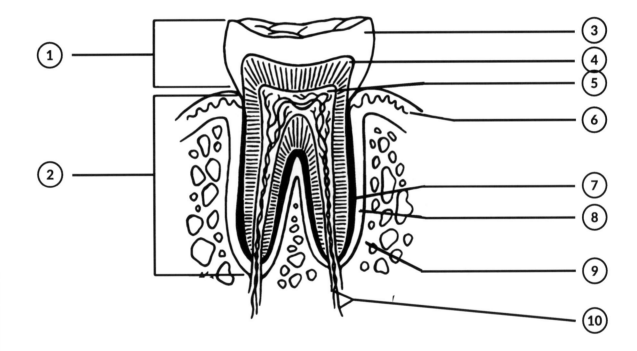

Tooth Anatomy

(1). Crown
(2). Root
(3). Enamel
(4). Dentin
(5). Pulp
(6). Gum
(7). Cementum
(8). Periodontal Membrane
(9). Bone
(10). Nerve And Blood Supply

Brain Anatomy

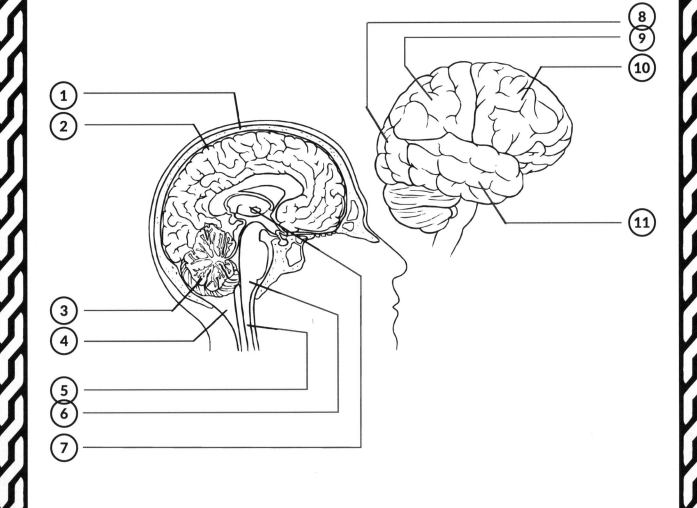

Brain Anatomy

(1). Cranium
(2). Corex
(3). Cerebellum
(4). Dura
(5). Spinal Cord
(6). Brain Stem
(7). Basal Ganglia
(8). Occipital Lobe
(9). Parietal Lobe
(10). Frontal Lobe
(11). Temporal Lobe

Human Body Diagram

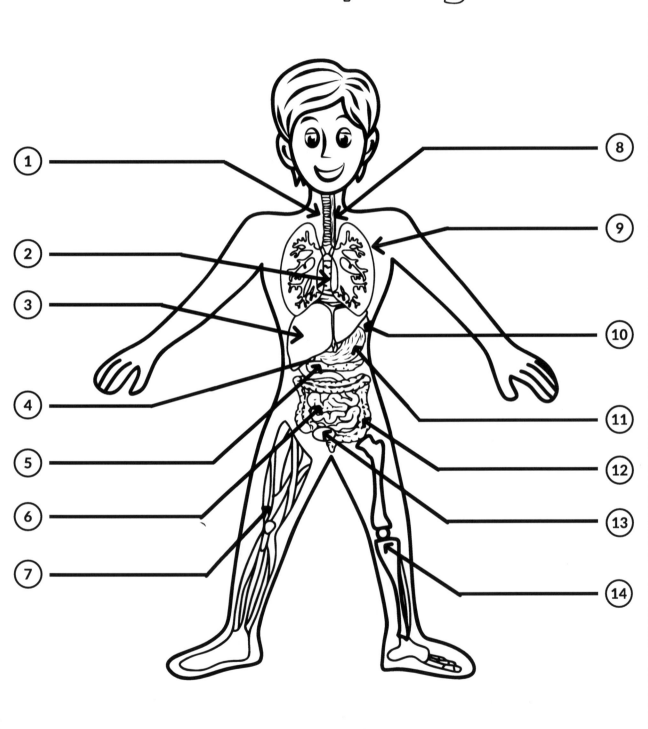

Human Body Diagram

(1). Trachea
(2). Heart
(3). Liver
(4). Gall Bladder
(5). Pancreas
(6). Small Intestine
(7). Muscle
(8). Esophagus
(9). Lungs
(10). Spleen
(11). Stomach
(12). Large Intestine
(13). Bladder
(14). Bone

Mouth and Pharynx

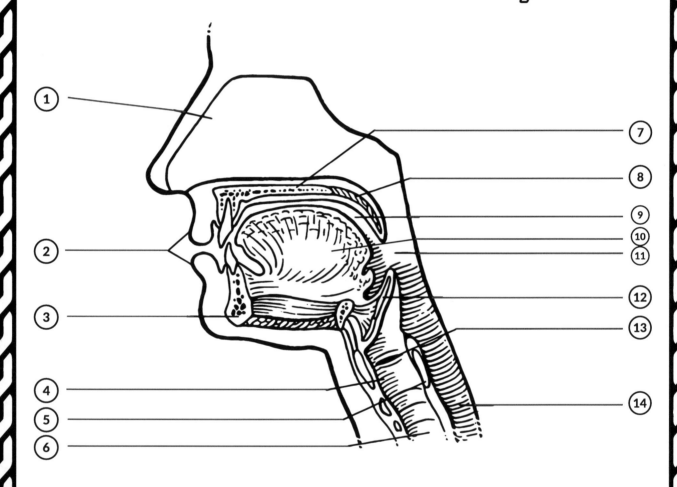

Mouth and Pharynx

(1). Nasal Cavity
(2). Lips
(3). Mandible
(4). Larynx
(5). Cricoid Cartilage
(6). Trachea (Windpipe)
(7). Hard Palate
(8). Soft Palate
(9). Oral Cavity
(10). Tongue
(11). Pharynx
(12). Epiglottis
(13). Vocal Fold
(14). Esophagus

Hand Anatomy

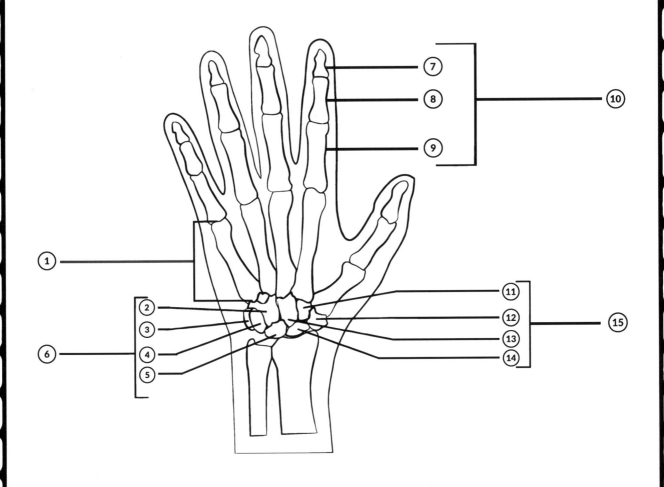

Hand Anatomy

(1). Metacarpal Bones
(2). Hamate
(3). Triquetrum
(4). Pisiform
(5). Lunate
(6). Carpal Bones
(7). Distal
(8). Middle
(9). Proximal
(10). Phalanges
(11). Trapezoid
(12). Trapezium
(13). Capitate
(14). Scaphoid
(15). Carpal Bones

Leg Anatomy

1. _____
2. _____
3. _____
4. _____
5. _____
6. _____
7. _____

Leg Anatomy

(1). Tarsals

(2). Metatarsals

(3). Phalanges

(4). Femur

(5). Patella

(6). Fibula

(7). Tibia

Foot Bones Anatomy

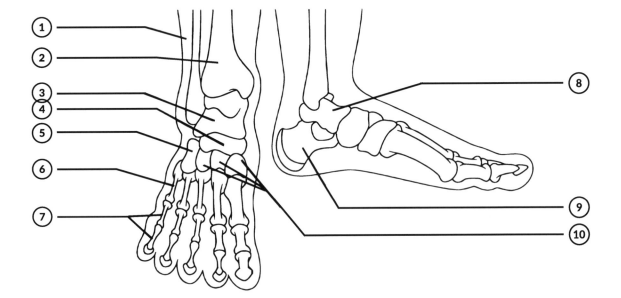

Foot Bones Anatomy

(1). Fibula
(2). Tibia
(3). Talus(Ankle Bone)
(4). Navicular
(5). Cuboid
(6). Metatarsals
(7). Phalanges
(8). Talus(Ankle Bone)
(9). Calcaneus (Heel Bone)
(10). Cuneiforms

Ear Anatomy

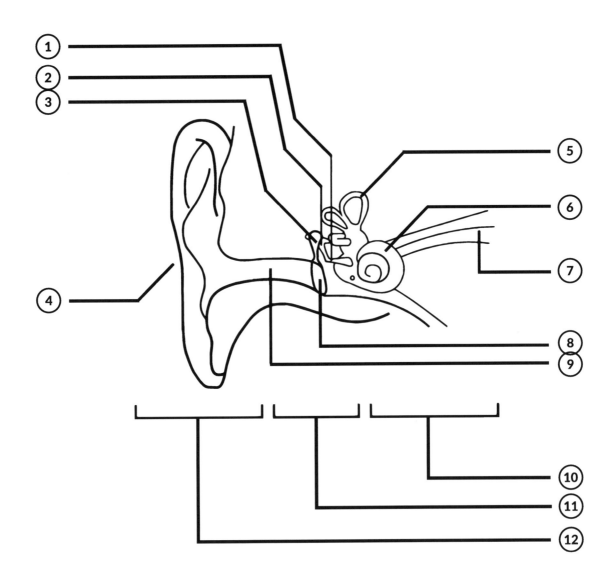

Ear Anatomy

(1). Stirrup
(2). Anvil
(3). Hammer
(4). Pinna
(5). Semicircular Canals
(6). Cochlea
(7). Auditory Nerve
(8). Ear Drum
(9). Auditory Canal
(10). Inner Ear
(11). Middle Ear
(12). Outer Ear

Pancreas Anatomy

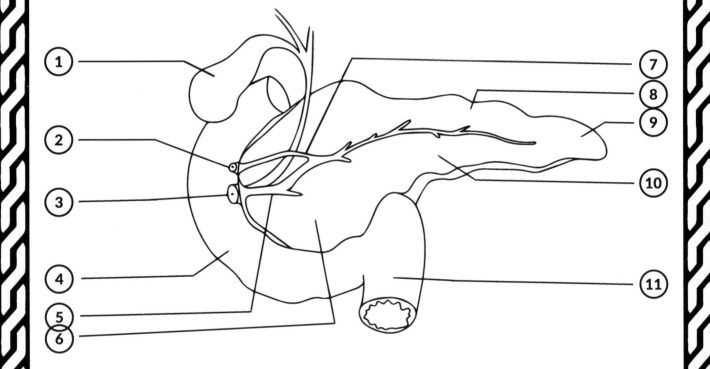

Pancreas Anatomy

(1). Gallbladder
(2). Minor Duodenal Papilla
(3). Major Duodenal Papilla
(4). Duodenum
(5). Main Pancreatic Duct
(6). Head
(7). Accessory Pancreatic Duct
(8). Pancreas
(9). Tail
(10). Body
(11). Jejunum

Stomach Anatomy

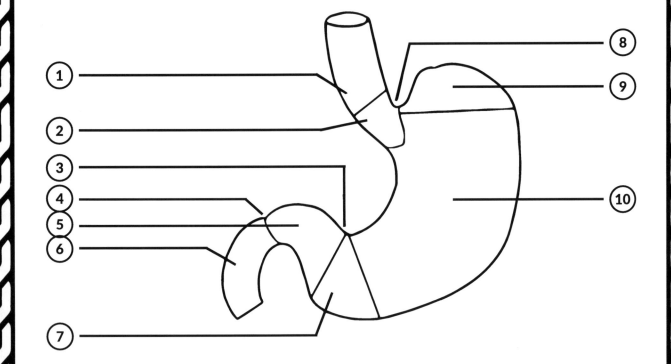

Stomach Anatomy

(1). Esophagus
(2). Cardia
(3). Angular Incisure
(4). Pylorus
(5). Pyloric Canal
(6). Duodenum
(7). Pyloric Antrum
(8). Cardiac Notch
(9). Fundus
(10). Body

Endocrine System

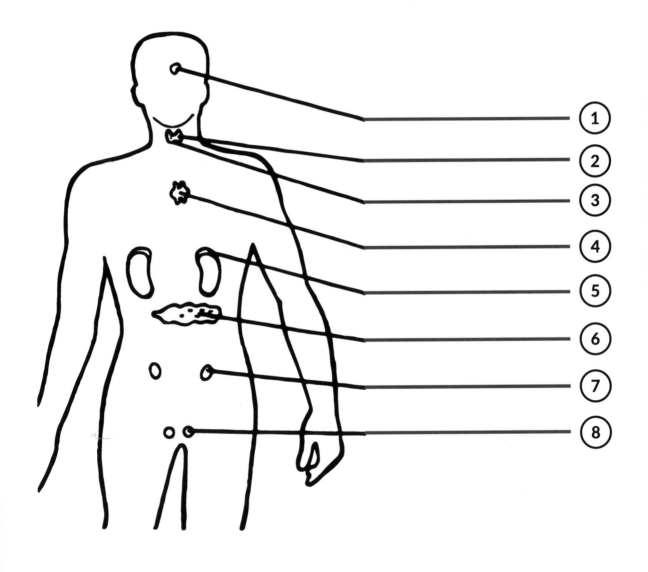

1. _____
2. _____
3. _____
4. _____
5. _____
6. _____
7. _____
8. _____

Endocrine System

(1). Pituitary Gland
(2). Parathyroid Glands
(3). Thyroid Gland
(4). Thymus Gland
(5). Adrenal Glands
(6). Island Of Langerhans
(7). Ovaries (Female)
(8). Testes (Male)

Urinary System

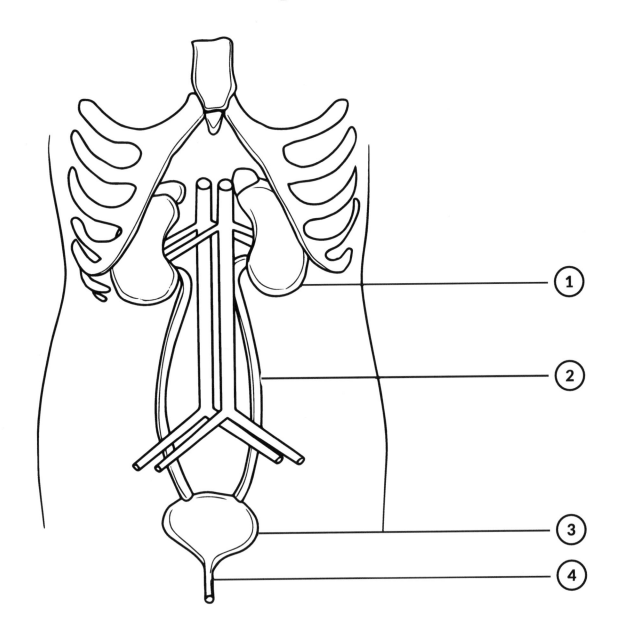

Urinary System
(1). Kidney
(2). Ureter
(3). Bladder
(4). Urethra

Head and Neck

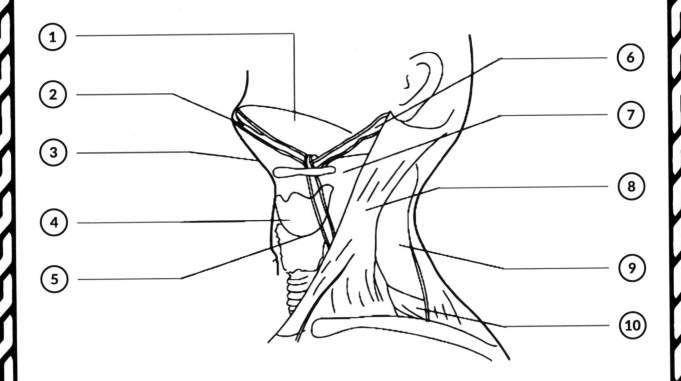

1.
2.
3.
4.
5.
6.
7.
8.
9.
10.

Head and Neck

(1). Submandibular Triangle
(2). Digastric Muscle
(3). Submental Triangle
(4). Muscular Triangle
(5). Omohyoid Muscle
(6). Digastric Muscle
(7). Carotid Triangle
(8). Sternocleidomastoid Muscle
(9). Lateral(Posterior) Triangle
(10). Omohyoid Muscle

Digestive System

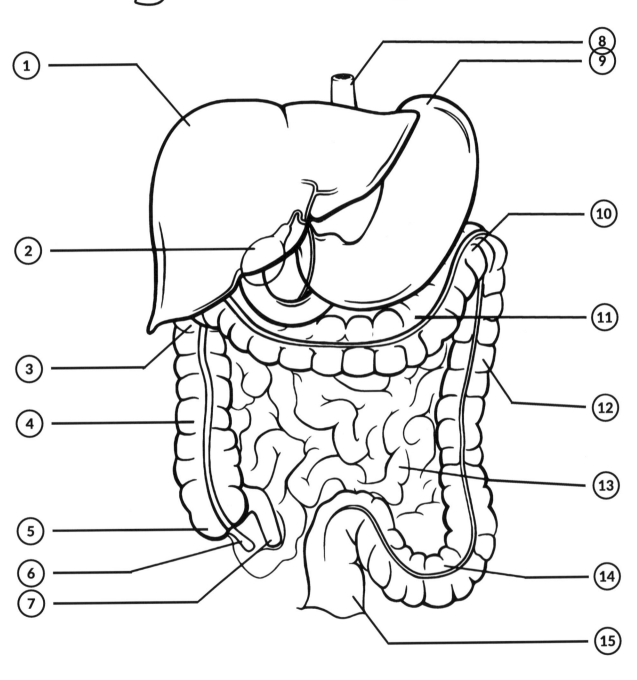

Digestive System

(1). Liver
(2). Gall Bladder
(3). Right Colic Flexure
(4). Ascending Colon
(5). Cecum
(6). Appendix
(7). Illeum
(8). Esophagus
(9). Stomach
(10). Left Colic Flexure
(11). Transverse Colon
(12). Decending Colon
(13). Small intestine
(14). Sigmoid Colon
(15). Rectum

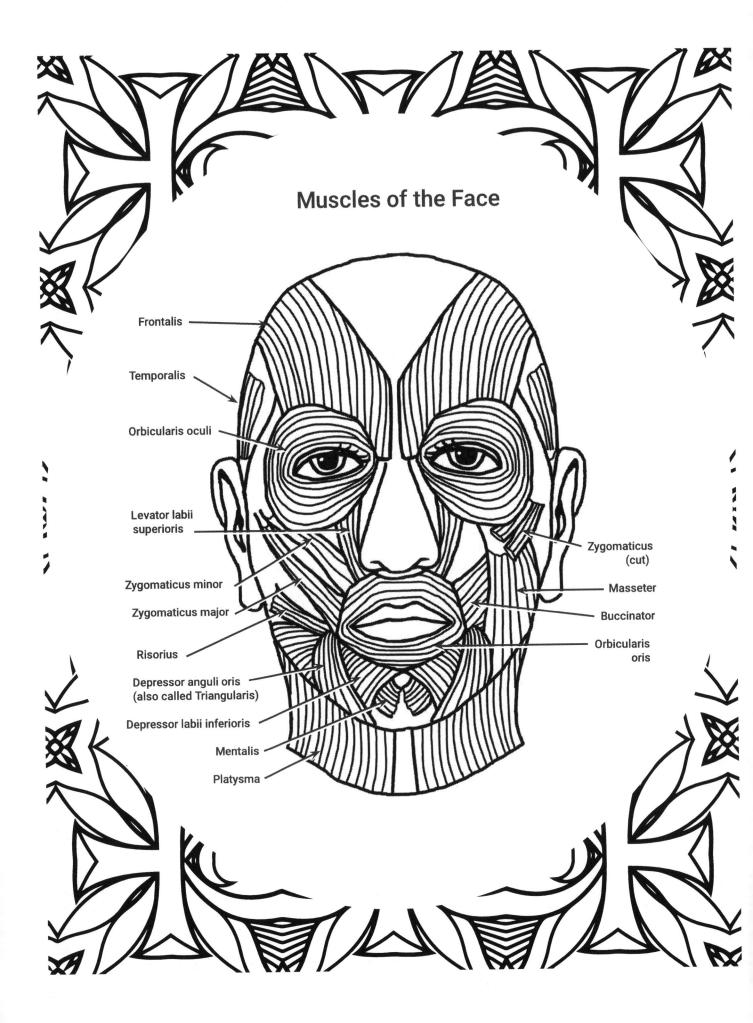

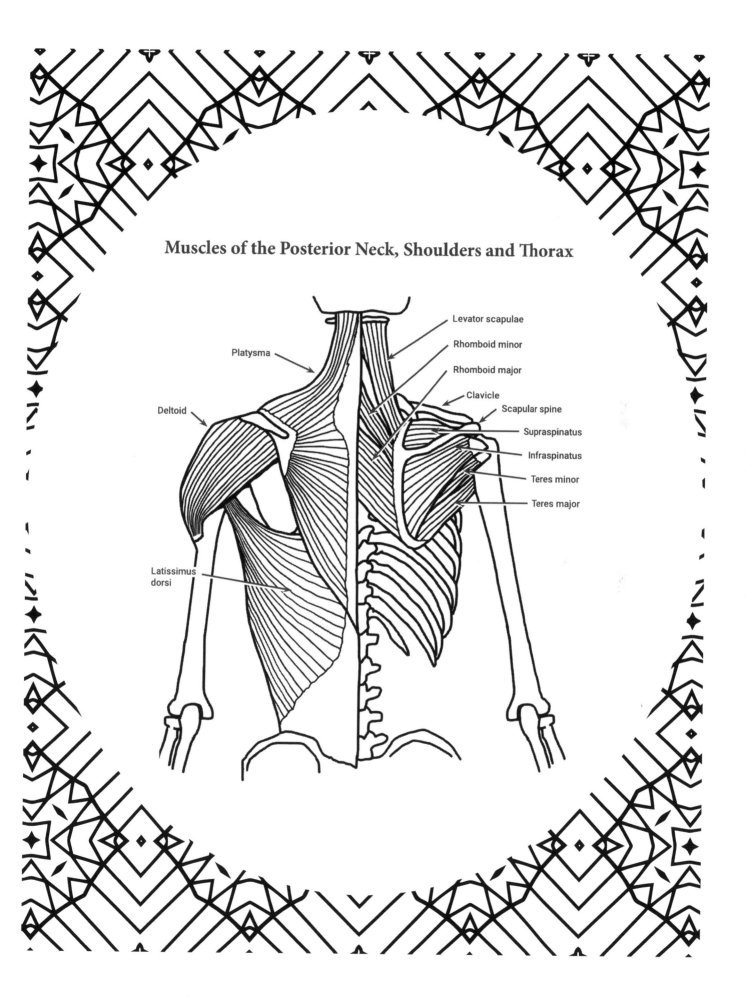

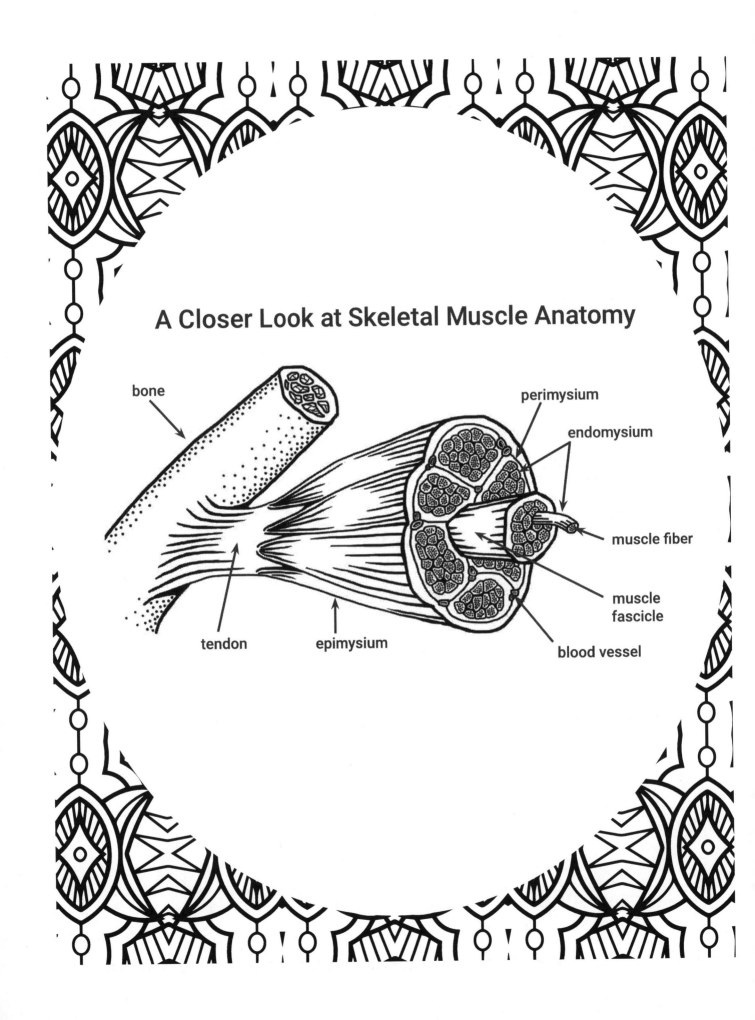

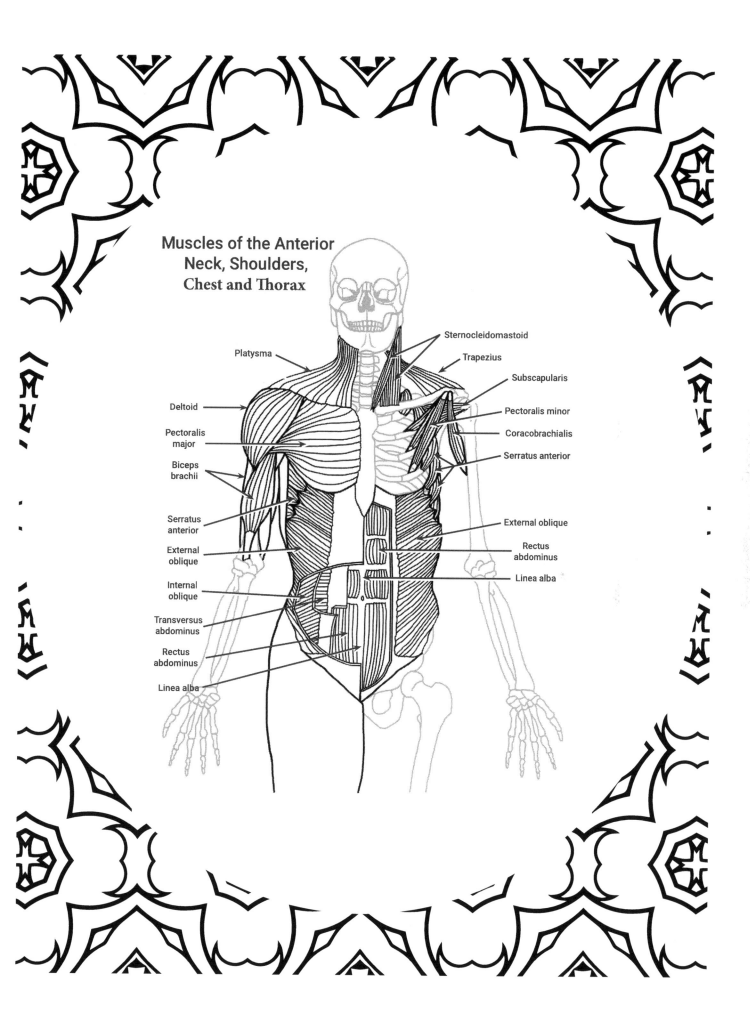

Muscles of Anterior Forearm

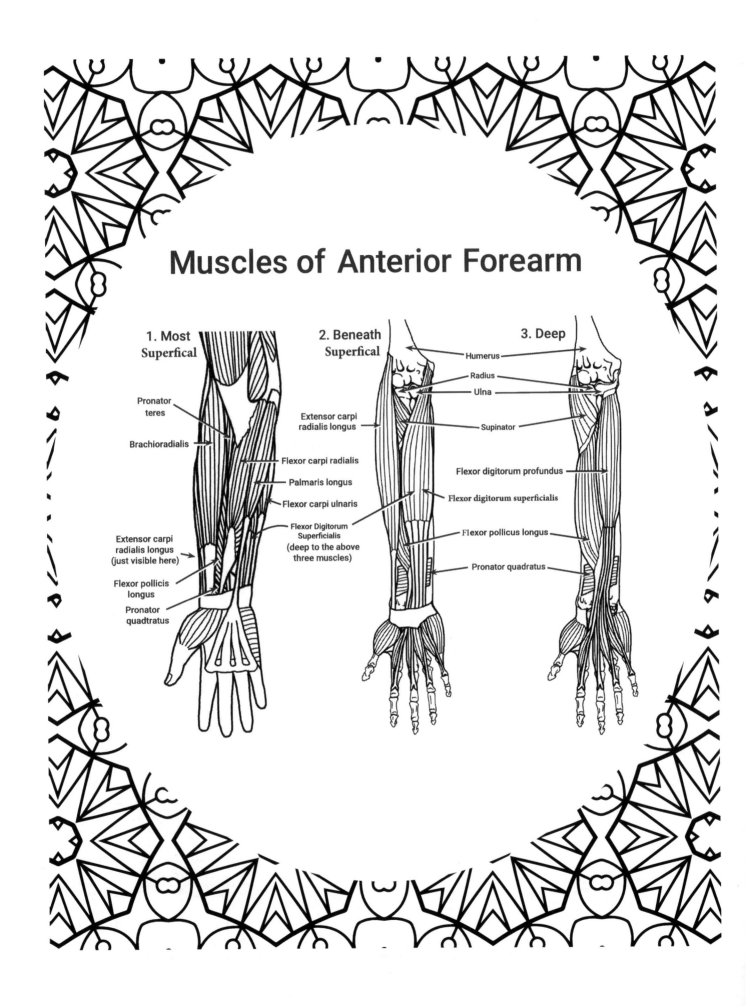

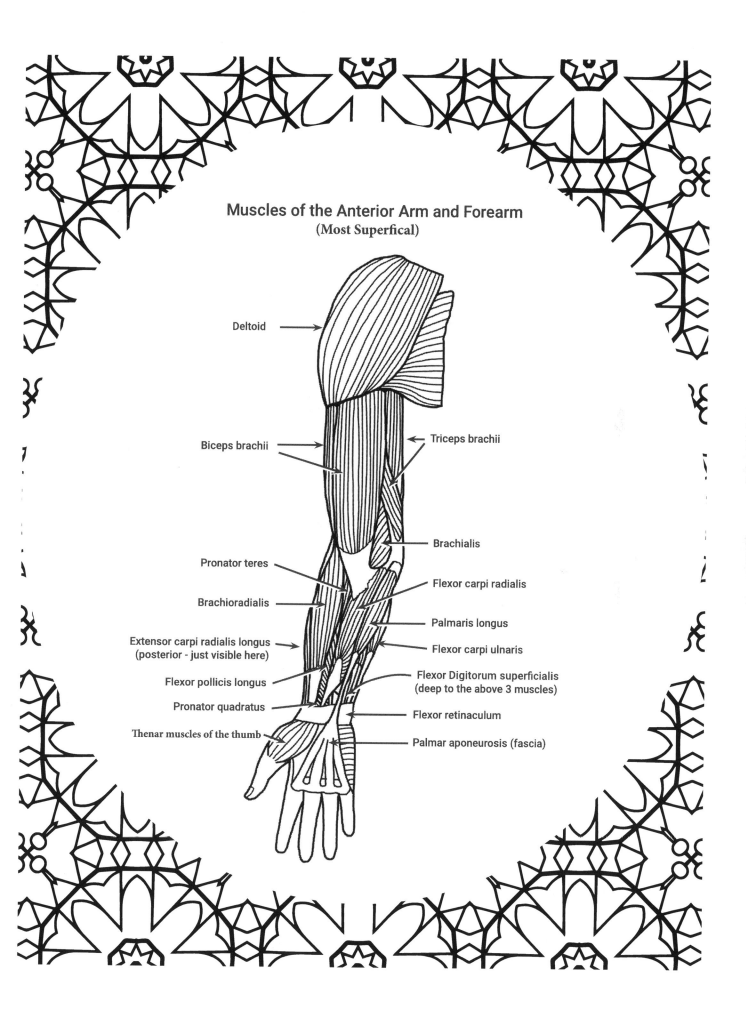

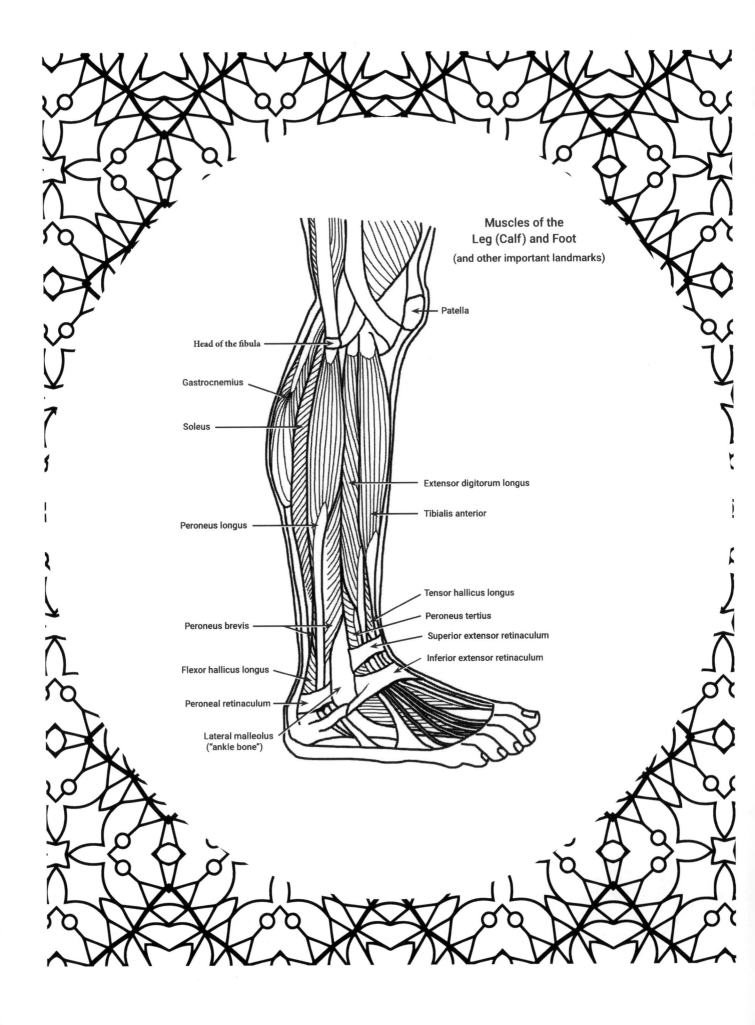

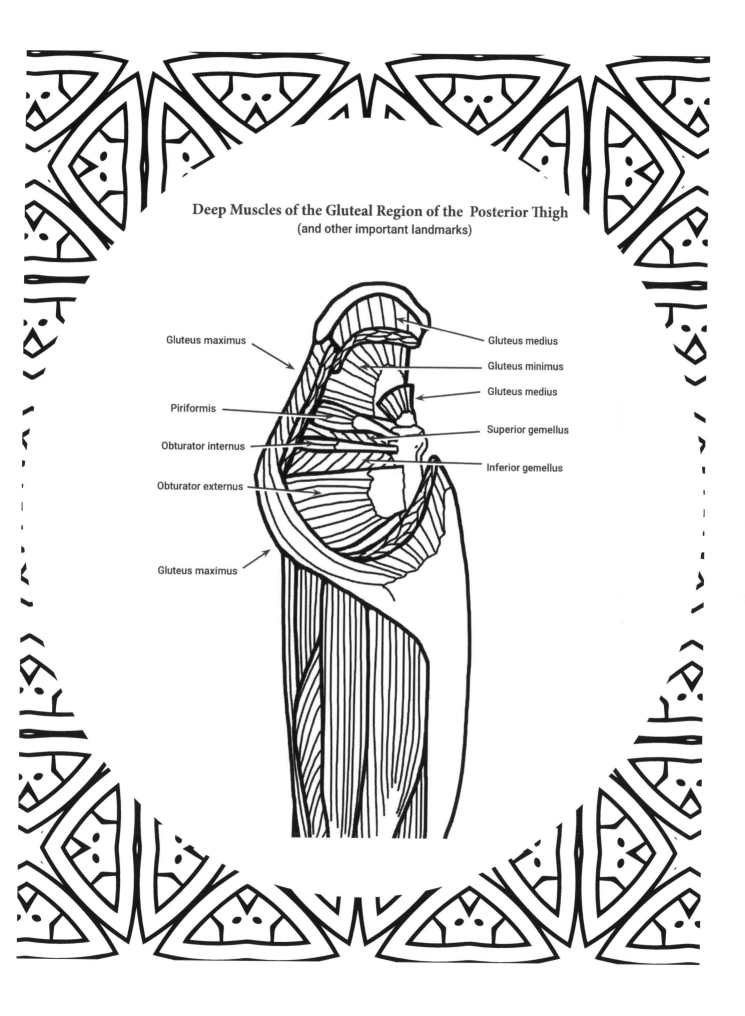

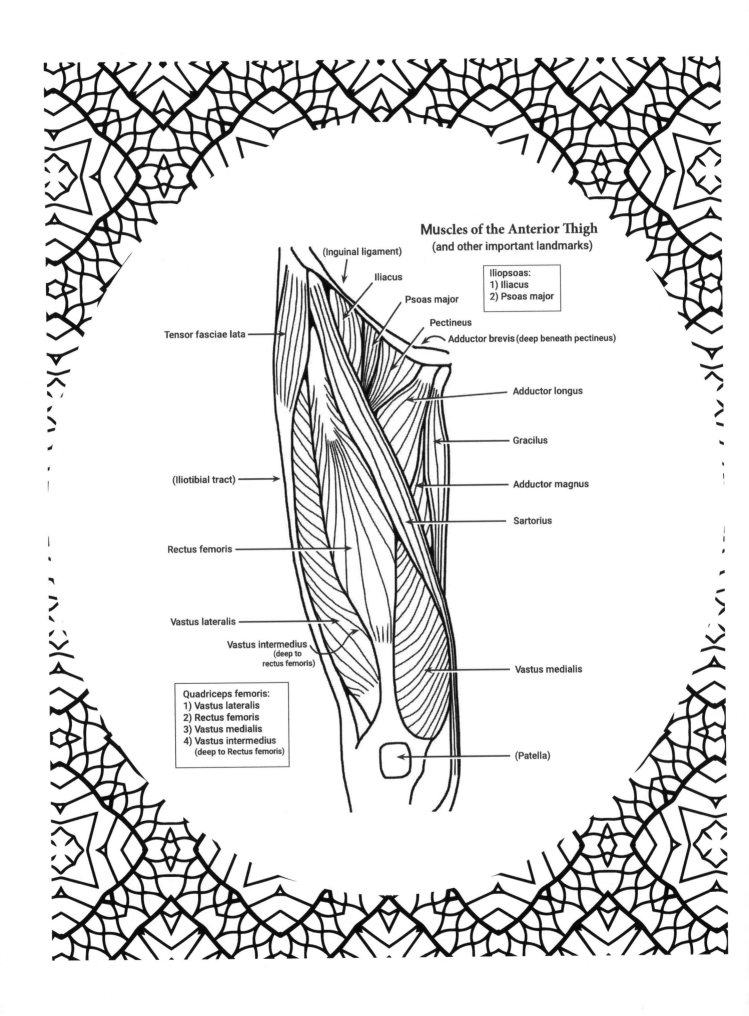

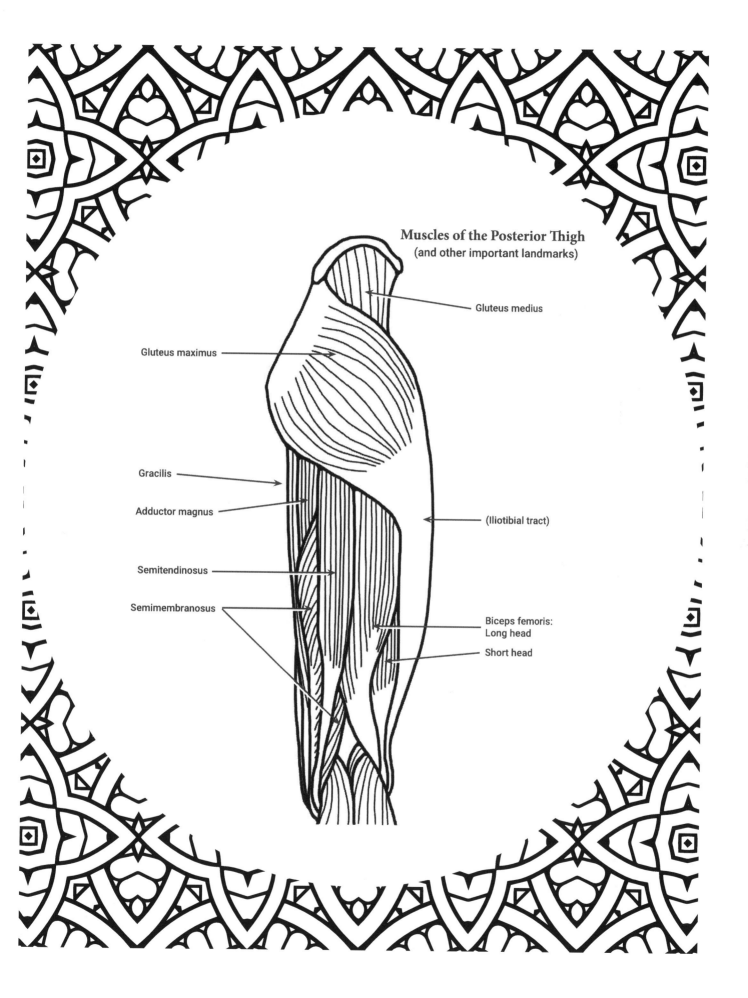

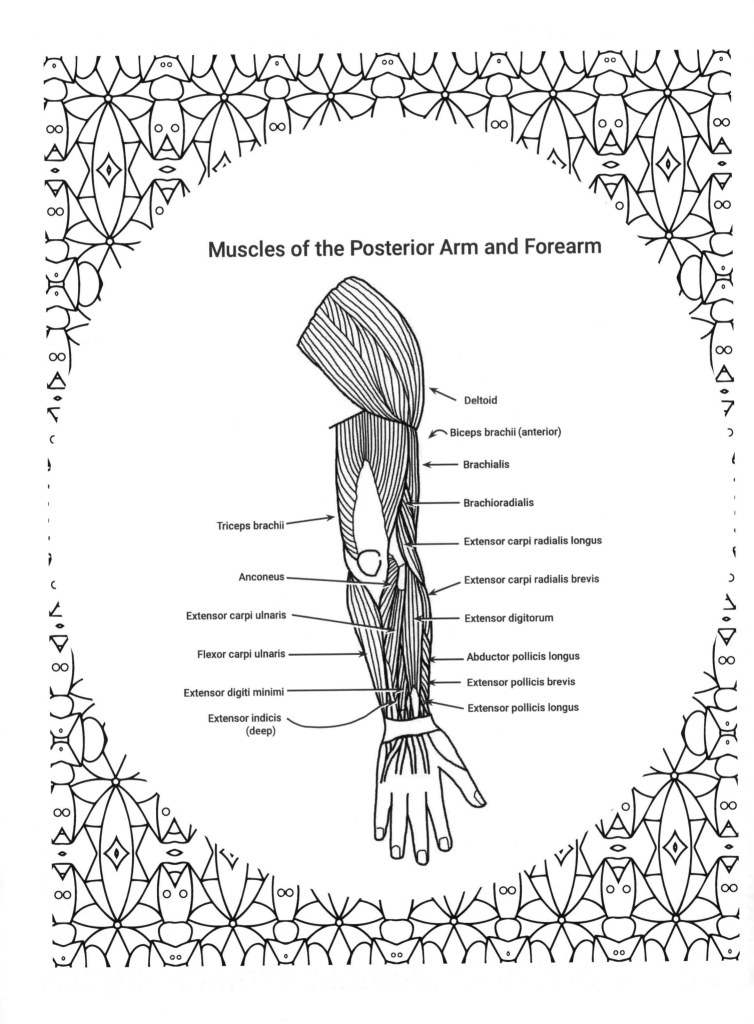

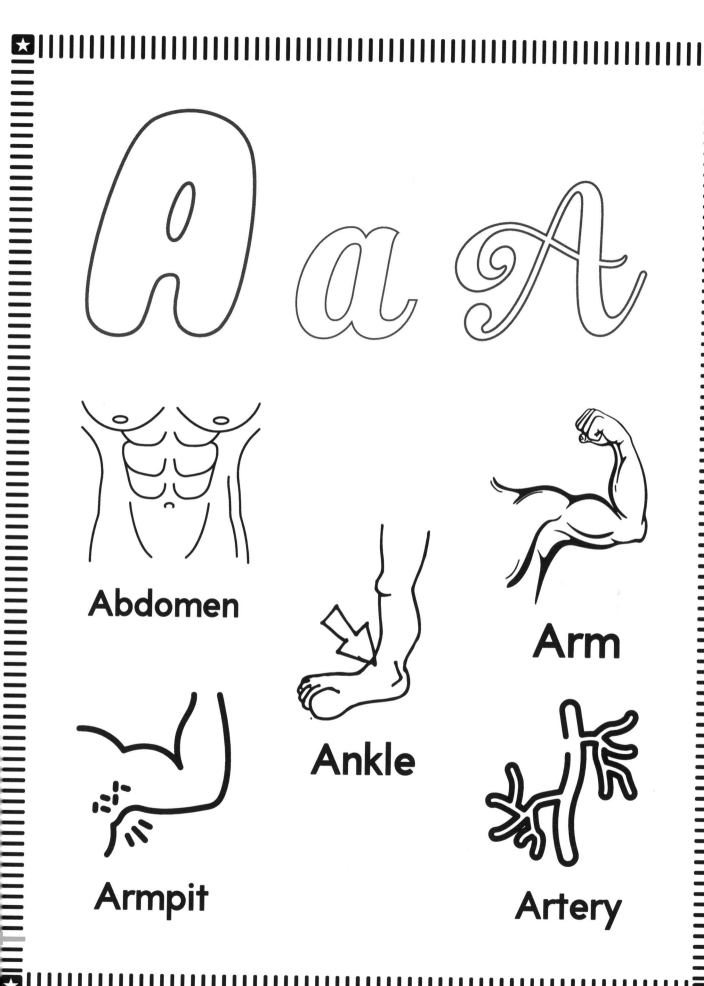

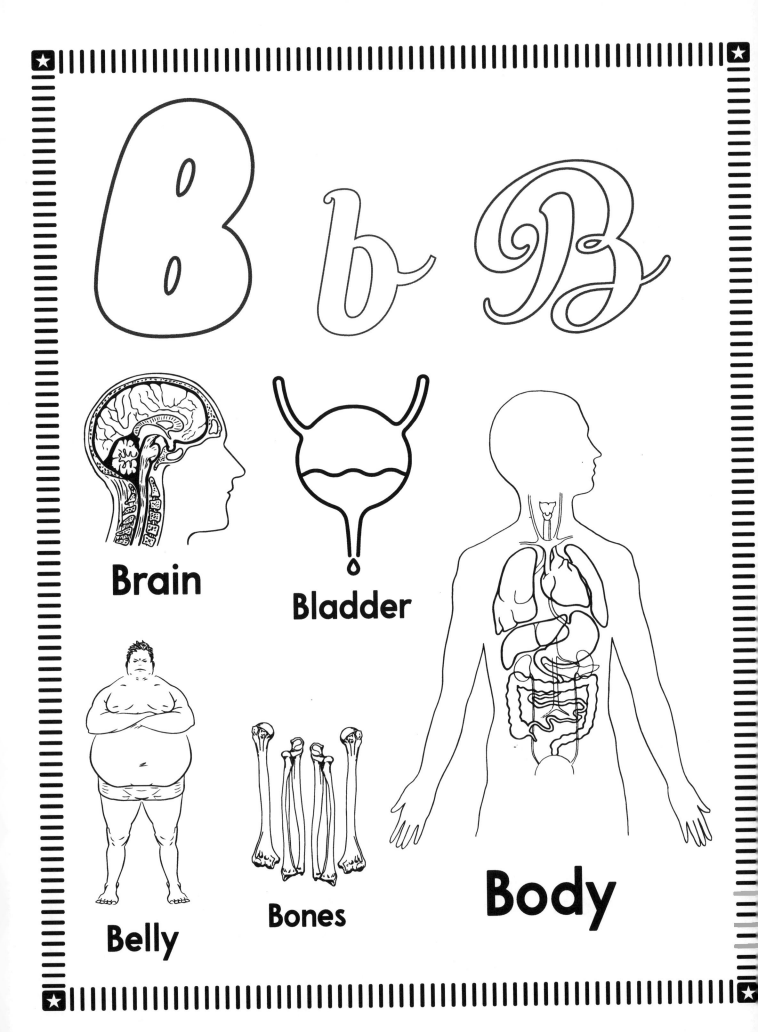

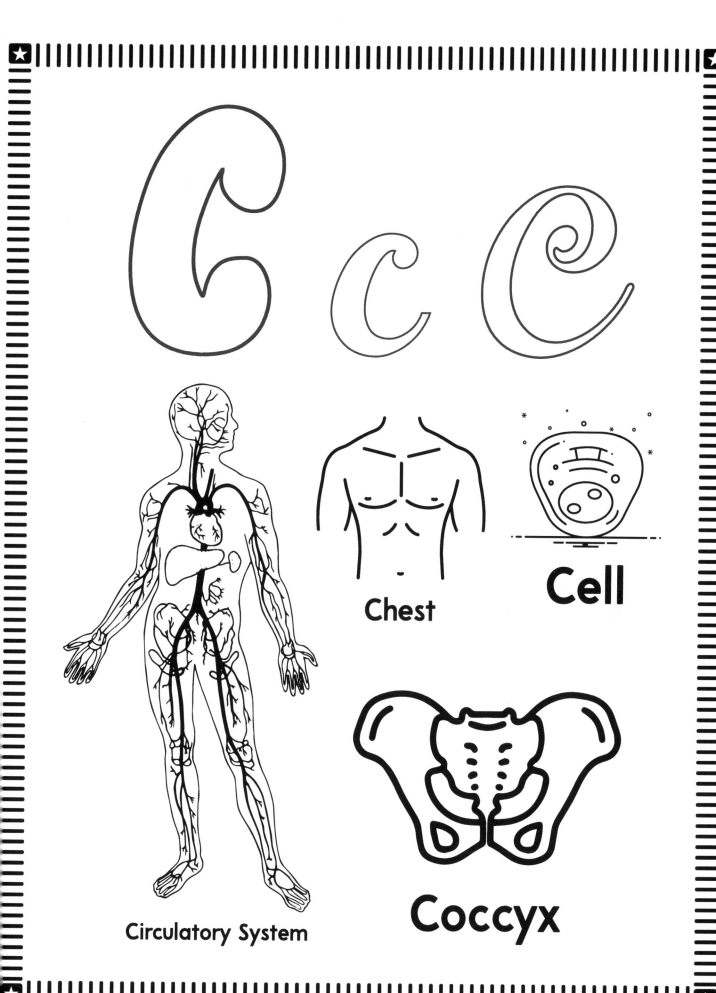

D d D

Digestive System

Dandruff

DNA

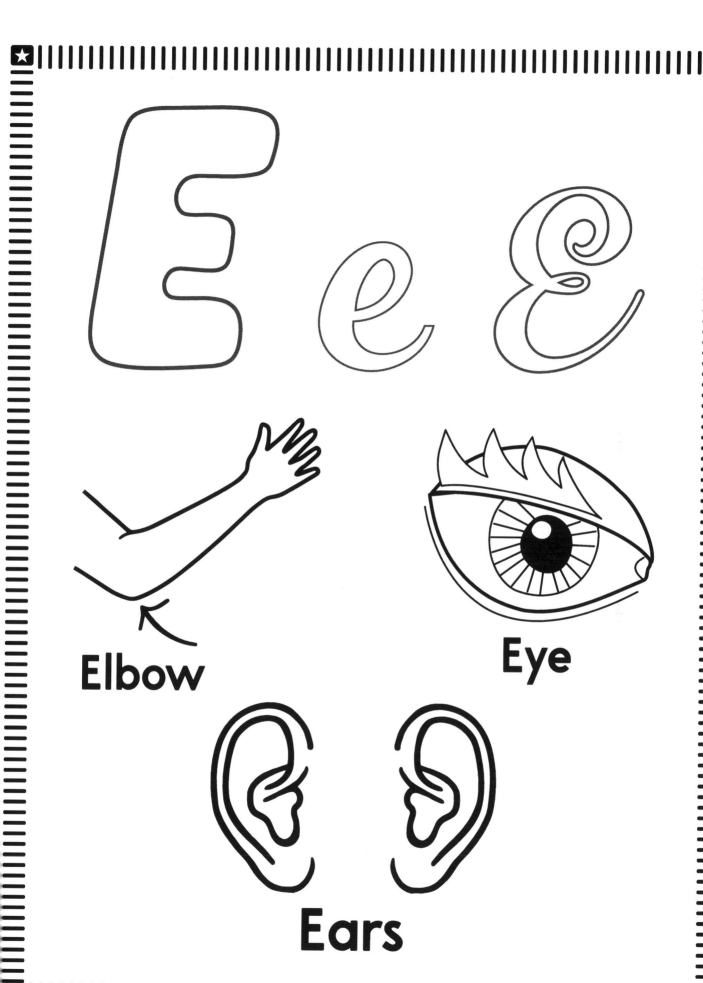

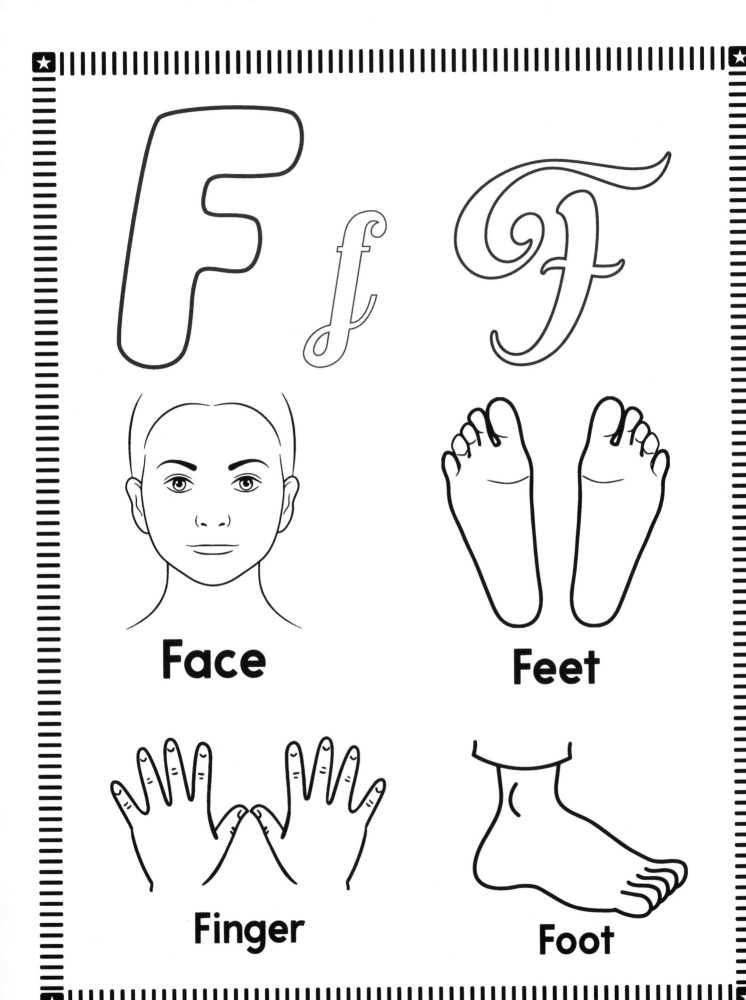

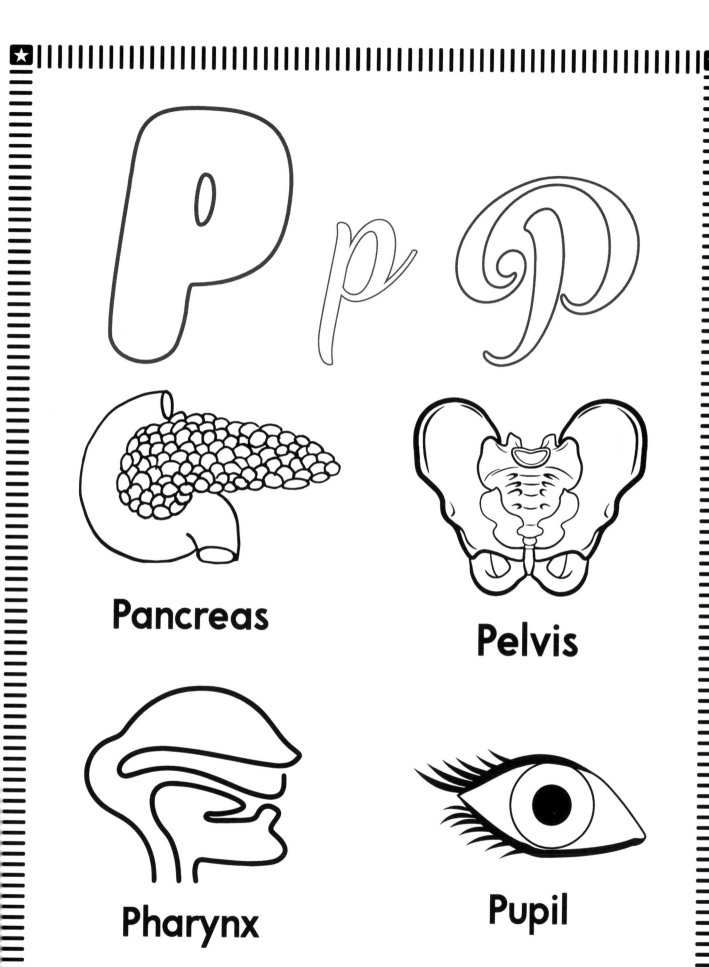

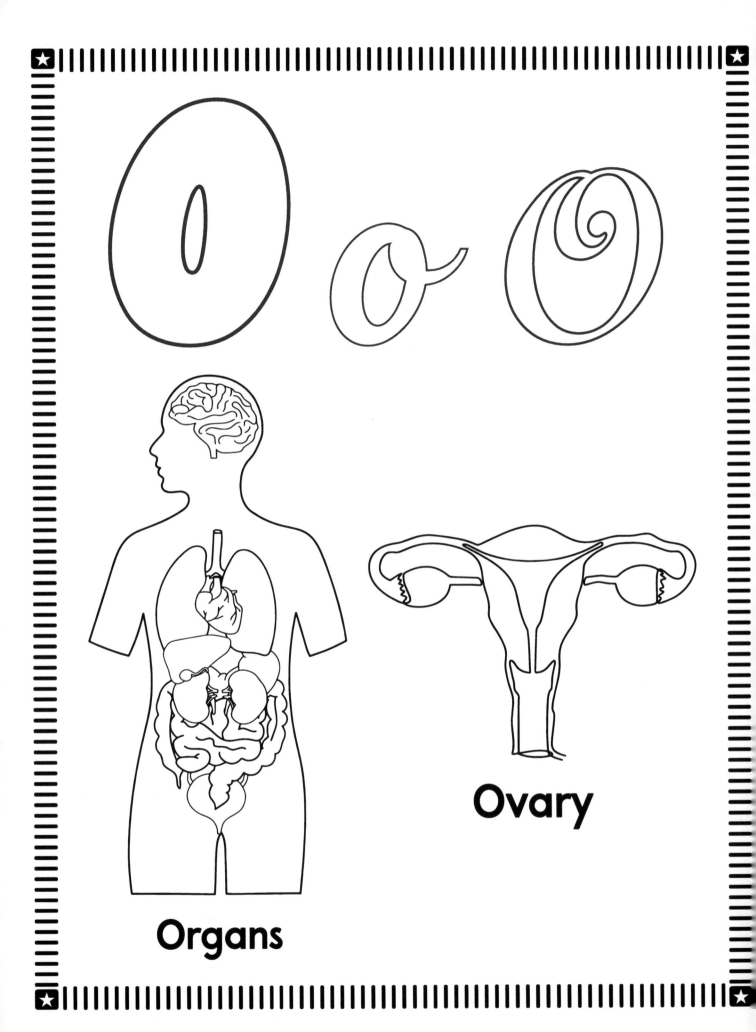

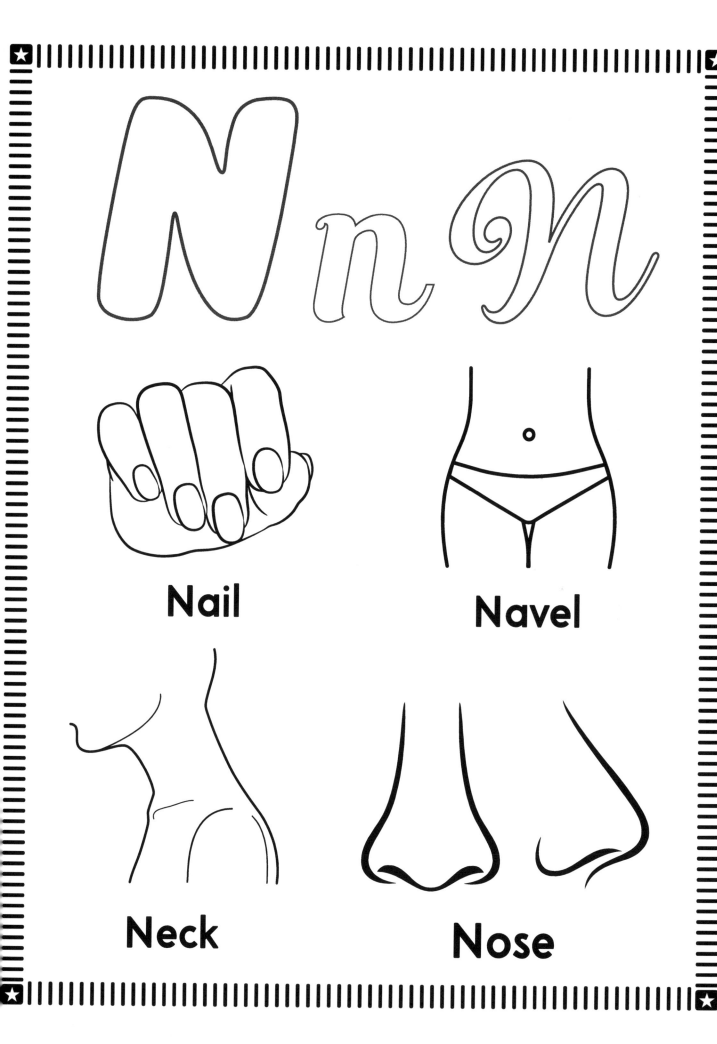

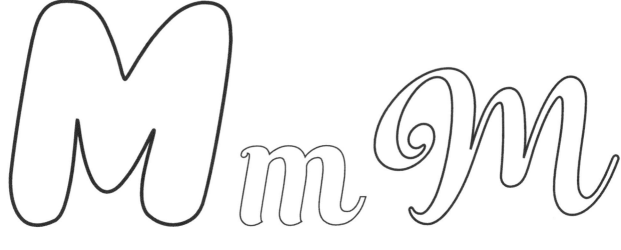

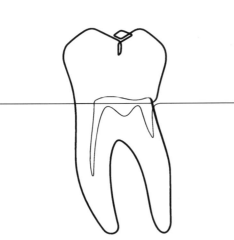
Molar

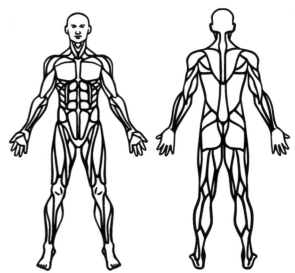
Muscles

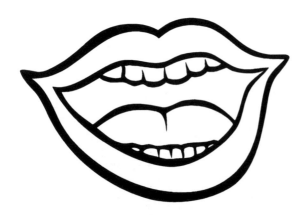
Mouth

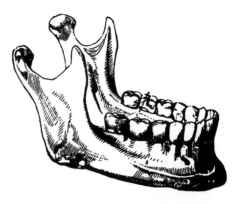
Mandible

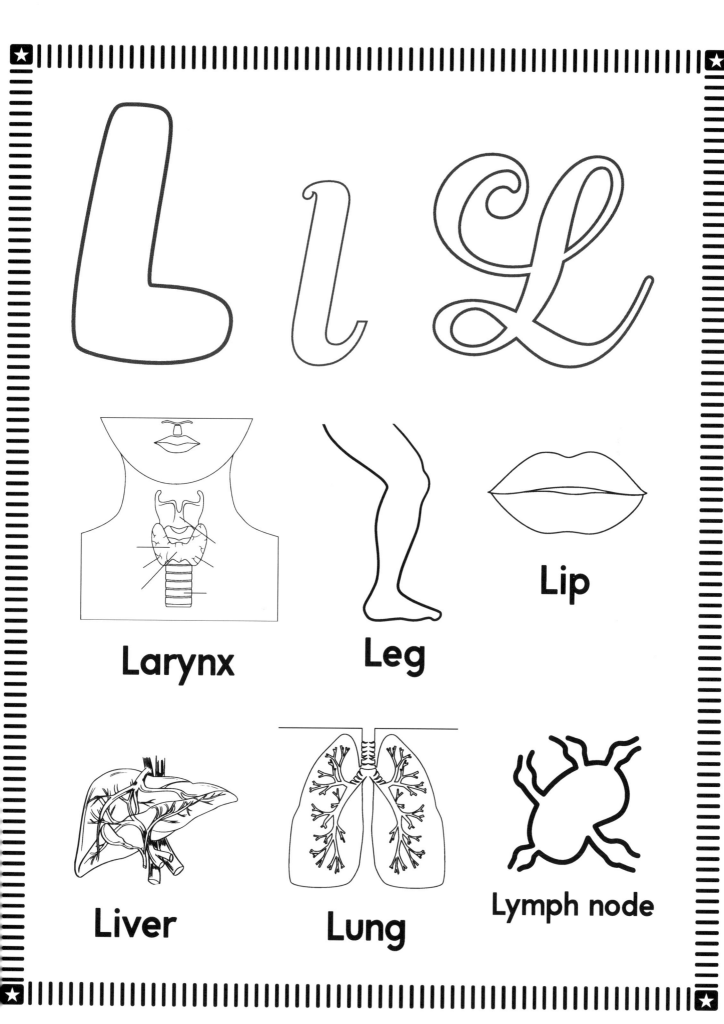

K k 𝒦

Kidney   **Knee**

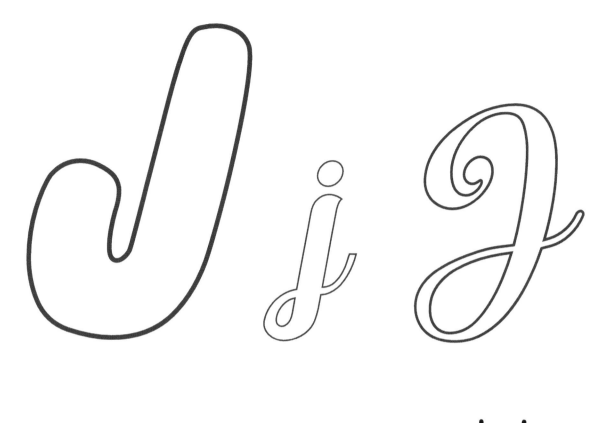

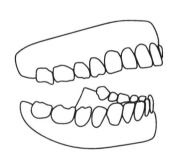 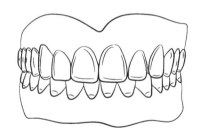 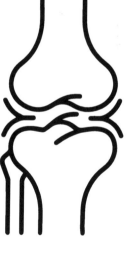

Jaws **Joint**

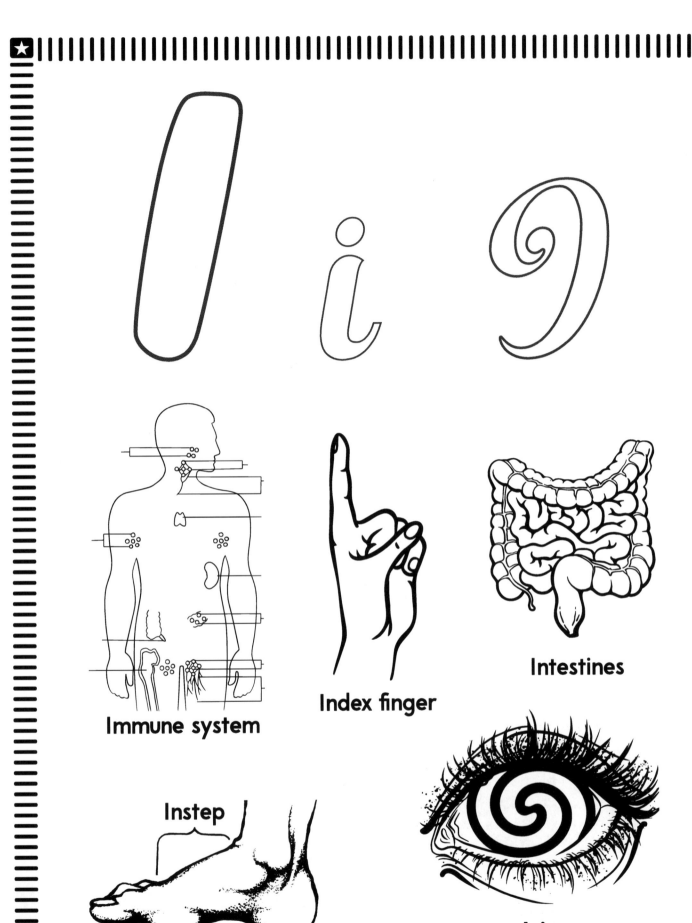

H h ℋ

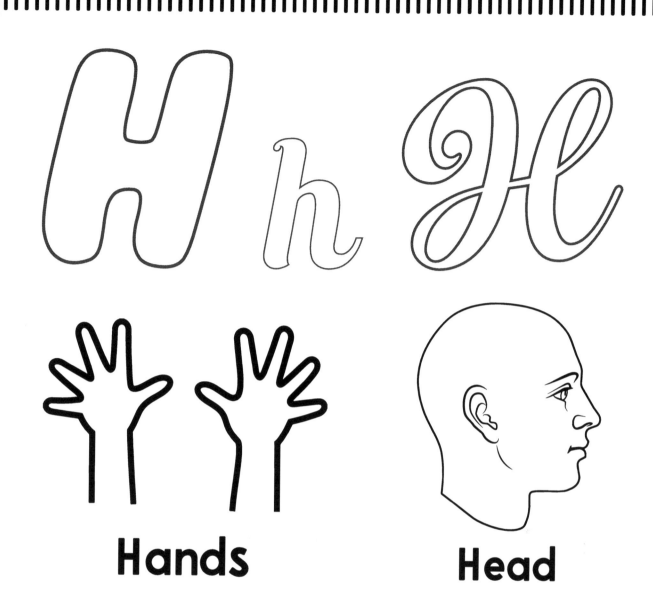

Hands **Head**

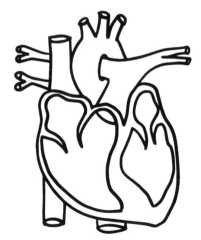
Heart

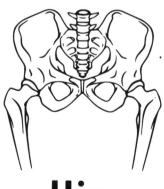
Hip

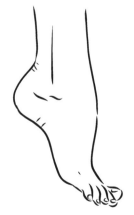
Heel

G g G

Gallbladder

Gland

Groin

Gum

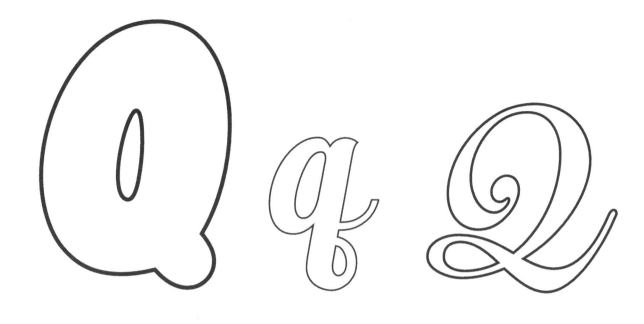

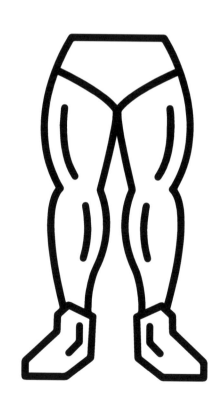
Quadriceps

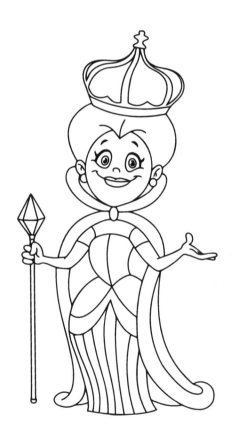
Queen

R r R

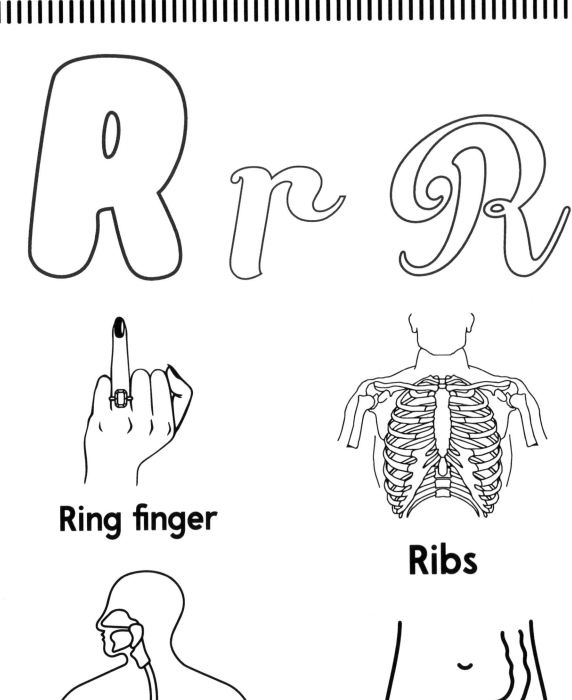

Ring finger

Ribs

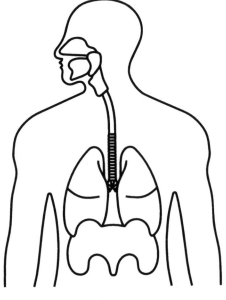

Respiratory Rystem

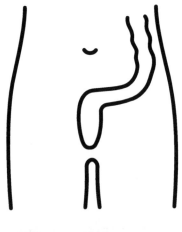

Rectum

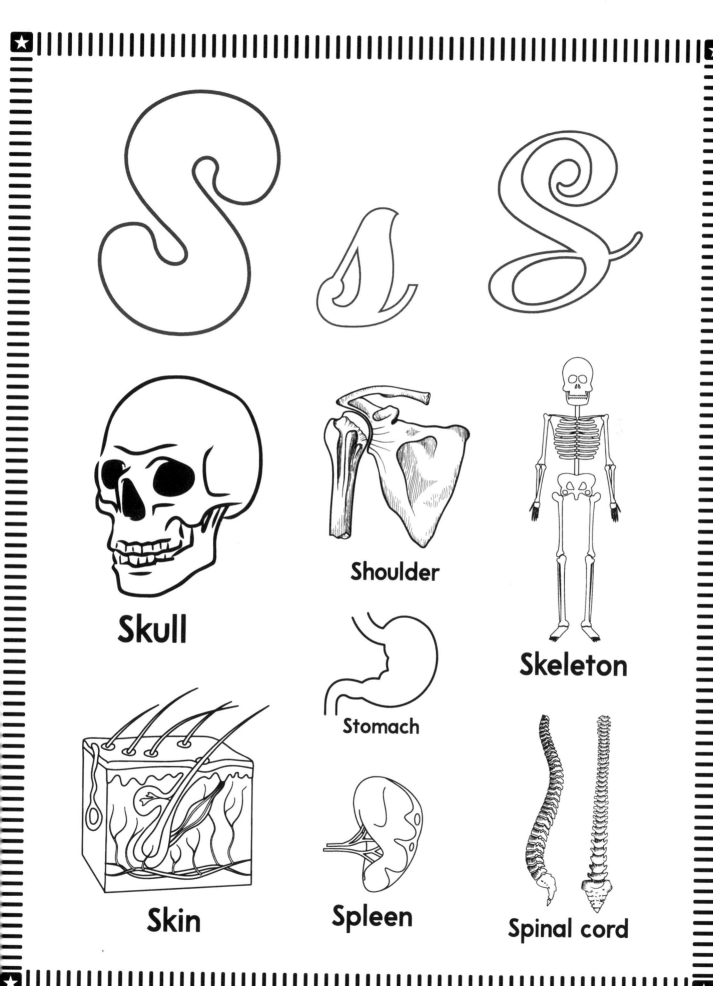

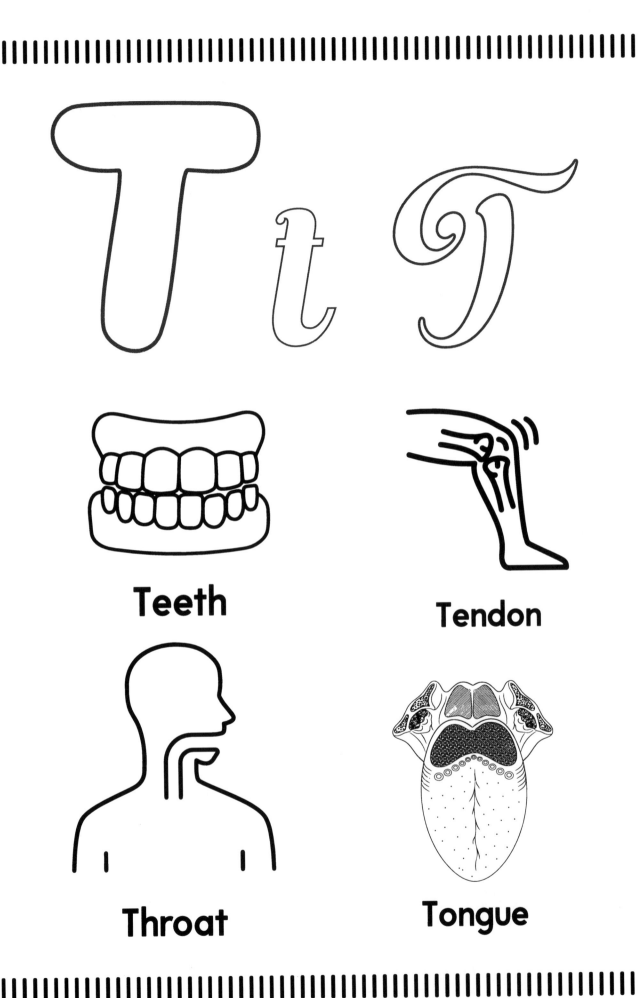

U u U

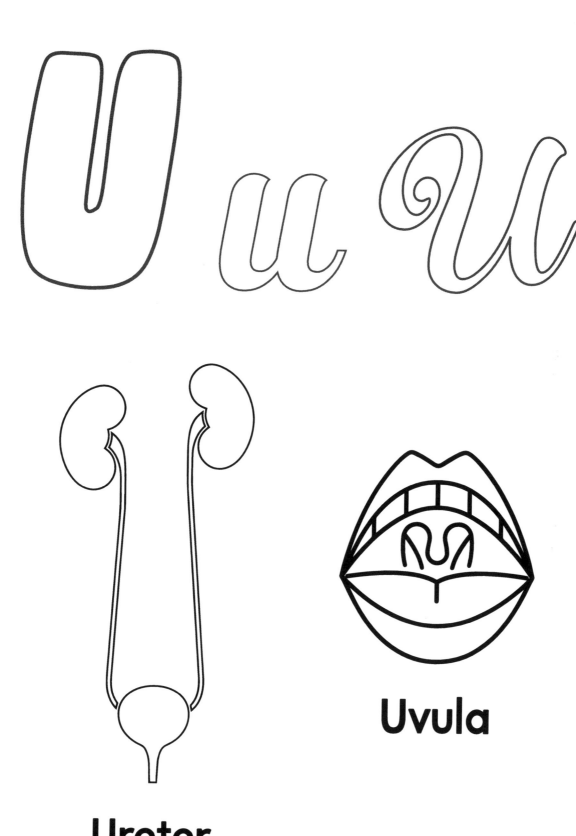

Ureter

Uvula

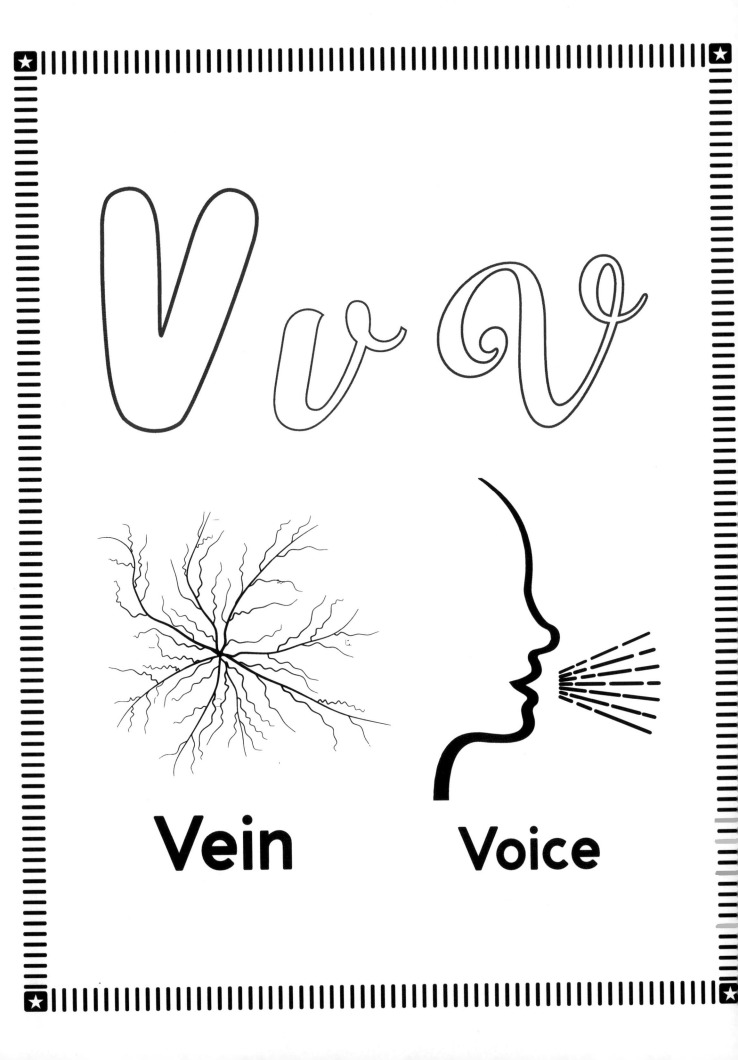

W w 𝒲

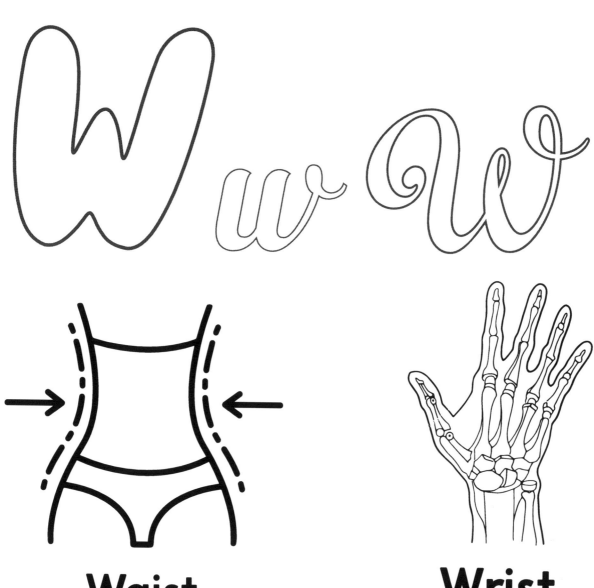

Waist

Wrist

White Blood Cell

Womb

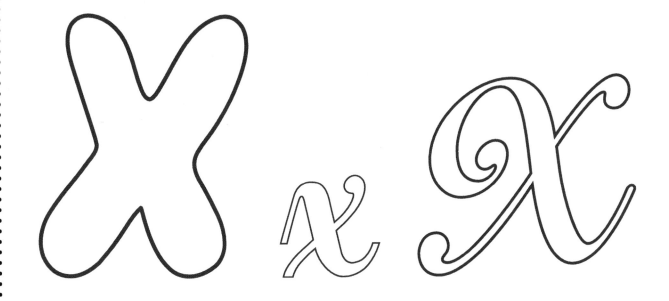

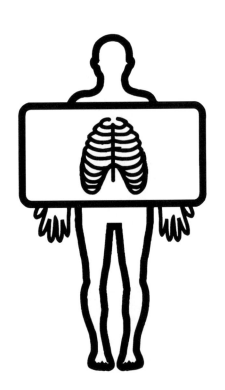 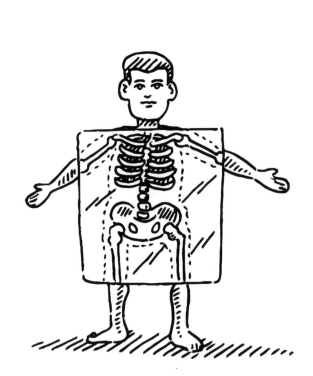

X-ray

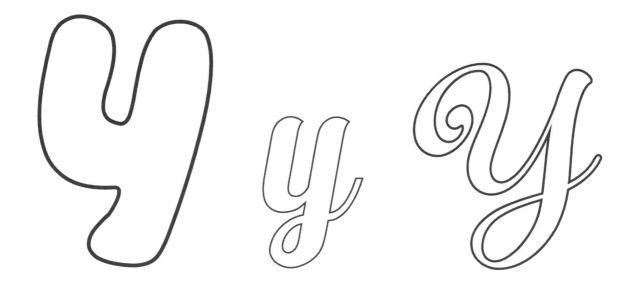

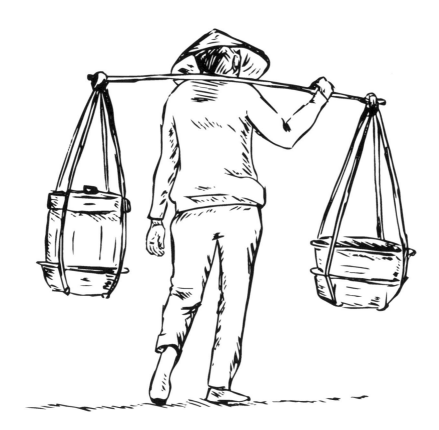

Yoke

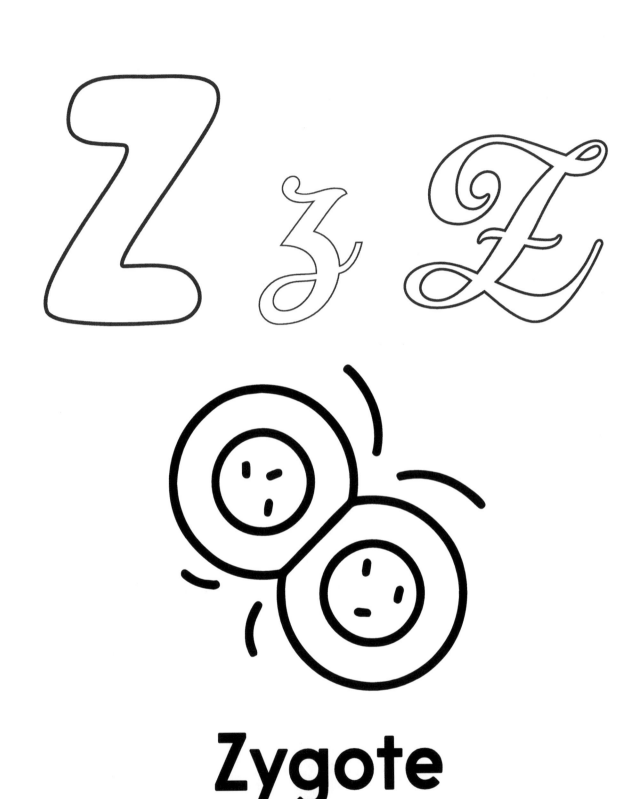

Zygote

Made in the USA
Columbia, SC
17 December 2021